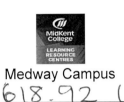

Trouble Talking

of related interest

**Language Development in Children
with Special Needs**
Performative Communication
Irene Johansson
ISBN 1 85302 241 1

Children with Language Impairments
An Introduction
Morag L Donaldson
ISBN 1 85302 313 2

Children with Special Needs
Assessment, Law and Practice –
Caught in the Acts, 3rd edition
John Friel
ISBN 1 85302 280 2

A Little Edge of Darkness
A Boy's Triumph Over Dyslexia
Tanya Faludy and Alexander Faludy
ISBN 1 85302 357 4

Trouble Talking

A guide for the parents of children with speech and language difficulties

James Law and Jane Elias

Jessica Kingsley Publishers
London and Bristol, Pennsylvania

The right of James Law and Jane Elias to be identified as authors of this work has been asserted by them in accordance with the Copyright, Designs and Patents Act 1988.

First published in the United Kingdom in 1996 by
Jessica Kingsley Publishers Ltd
116 Pentonville Road
London N1 9JB, England
and
1900 Frost Road, Suite 101
Bristol, PA 19007, U S A

Copyright © 1996 James Law and Jane Elias

Library of Congress Cataloging in Publication Data
Law, James (lecturer),
Trouble talking : a guide for parents of children with
difficulties communicating / James Law and Jane Elias.
p.   cm.
Includes bibliographical references and index.
ISBN 1-85302-253-5 (pbk. : alk. paper)
1. Language disorders in children–Popular works. I. Elias,
Jane 1955-
RJ496.L35L393   1996   96-22208
618.92'855–dc20   CIP

British Library Cataloguing in Publication Data
Law, James
Trouble Talking:Guide for Parents of
Children with Difficulties Communicating
I. Title II. Elias, Jane
618.92855

ISBN 1-85302-253-5

Printed and Bound in Great Britain by
Cromwell Press, Melksham, Wiltshire

Contents

Introduction   1

1 Parents Talking   4

2 Getting Started: The Development of Speech and Language   18

3 The Assessment: What are Speech and Language Therapists
   Looking for?   34

4 What Else Can He Do? The View of Other Professionals   52

5 Labels and Diagnoses: What Happens After Assessment   74

6 Issues Commonly Associated with Speech and Language
   Difficulties   88

7 What Can We Do About It? Educational Provision   104

8 What Can We Do About It? Different Approaches to
   Intervention   117

9 What Can We Do About It? The Role of the Independent
   Sector   135

10 The Law and the Language-Impaired Child
   Sheila Denney   147

Useful books   157

Useful addresses   159

Appendix 1   161

Appendix 2   165

Glossary   168

Index   176

Dedication

To all the parents and children who
helped us write this book.

Introduction

The way that we learn to speak is a mysterious process. Most of us take it for granted and quickly forget how we acquired what is probably the most complex skill that we will ever come to learn. In the same way most parents take the development of language in their child for granted. It simply happens. We may laugh when our children first use their own sentences. We may feel embarrassed when they copy something we have said when we might have preferred they had not. We may correct a mispronunciation or a grammatical mistake as they get older. But for the most part we are simply spectators and partners in an extraordinary and fascinating process.

Whilst most children find this effortless, for some it is altogether much more complicated and confusing. They are slow in starting to speak or, when they do start, what they say is very limited or unclear. In such cases parents often come to think more clearly about the process of acquisition, so that they can understand what their child is experiencing and, of course, do as much as they can to help. This often leads to all sorts of questions about language: how we learn it, what goes wrong and what can be done about it. All too often parents say that when they want to speak to someone about it the right person is never around and by the time they do manage to see them the moment has passed.

This book is for parents who have children with speech and language difficulties. It is intended to help you answer your questions whether they be about language development in general, about what professionals are looking for when they assess children, what sort of difficulties your children are experiencing now, how they are likely to change as they grow older and about what sort of services are available to help them. The book is designed to allow you to ask these questions at your own speed. This last point is important because it is often difficult to take in all the information that is given when faced with a professional who knows the subject inside out but who does not know where you, the parent, are starting from in your own understanding.

The aim of the book is to allow you, the parent, to know what to expect from your children and from the services that are set up to provide for children with speech and language difficulties. In some ways this is an impossible task because every child is different and every health and education authority provides a different range of services. Nevertheless, we have learned much about these children over the last few years, and it is essential that you have access to the information available. It is only then that you can make informed decisions about the needs of your child.

This book is not designed to show you what to do with your child. Children differ so much one from another that making specific recommendations without knowing the child would be impossible. We have listed some useful texts at the end which may give you some ideas but really there is no substitute for speaking about your child with someone who both knows your child's needs well and who specialises in speech and language difficulties.

The book begins with a discussion of some of the most important issues from the parent's perspective. We hope that this will be helpful to those of you who feel that they are the only ones who have children who are experiencing difficulties in this area. Chapter 2 is devoted to a discussion of the way that speech and language development progresses from birth through to the school years. We then go on to show what different professionals look for when they are assessing children with difficulties acquiring language. We begin with the speech and language therapist (in Chapter 3) and go on to include the psychologist, the paediatrician and both occupational therapist and physiotherapist (in Chapter 4). In Chapter 5 we look at the process of diagnosis and the description of language in children with difficulties. Parents are often frustrated with what appears to be a bewildering array of terms used by different professionals. We then turn, in Chapter 6, to look at what we know about the natural course of language development in children who are experiencing difficulties in this area. The difficulties are sometimes discussed as if they occur on their own, but as any parent knows, difficulties in one area have all sorts of implications for other aspects of development.

We then go on to look at what can be done for these children. An overview of the different services available is provided in Chapter 7 and a more detailed look at the type of interventions commonly used is given in Chapter 8. In Chapter 9 we have included an overview of the contribution made by the independent sector notably the work of the charities, the Association For All Speech Impaired Children (AFASIC) and Invalid Children's Aid Nationwide (ICAN). In extreme cases parents may find themselves in a position of having recourse to the law to ensure that the necessary services are provided for their child. This process is discussed in Chapter 10 by Sheila Denney, a member of the Institute of Legal Executives who has considerable experience in this area. The book ends with a list of useful addresses, a summary of the stages of identification and assessment of Special Educational Needs, a glossary describing some technical terms you may come across and finally an index to help you look up issues that are important to you.

Such a book cannot hope to be exhaustive but we will have succeeded if we have given you a sound understanding of the issues concerned so that you can go on to become partners with the professionals providing the service.

In the process of preparing this book we have received help from a great many people. In particular we would like to mention the parents who contributed to Chapter 1 and those who looked at parts of the draft. Likewise we would like to thank colleagues, especially Jeanette Webb and Susie Summers who have commented on parts of the book at various stages. A number of other colleagues, Suzi Dummett for the cartoons, Shantal Baker for her administrative help and those who have helped us by writing specific parts of the book. We would like to thank the paediatrician, Sundara Lingam, the educational psychologist, Roger Penniceard, the physiotherapist, Sally Holt, and the occupational therapists, Liz Mathew and Ana Santo, for their contributions. We are equally indebted to Brian Jones and Fraser Mackay from Invalid Children Nationwide (ICAN) and Norma Corkish, Director of the Association for All Speech Impaired Children (AFASIC) for their contributions to the chapter on the independent sector. Finally we would like to thank Sheila Denney for giving the very up-to-date interpretation of the current legal position regarding language impaired children.

Jane Elias
James Law
1994

CHAPTER 1

Parents Talking

There has been a tendency for professionals to tell parents what they should think about the provision that their children need. This may be understandable because these professionals are bound to have opinions as to what is most likely to meet the needs of the children concerned. However, the people who have the greatest vested interest in the right decision are always the parents. But how do we know what parents' views are?

This chapter is made up of the responses of a number of parents to a set of questions about their children's needs. We have made use of our own questionnaire and where appropriate combined the results with those from a survey carried out by the Association for All Speech Impaired Children (see list of helpful texts at the end of this book). The children all had marked speech and/or language problems. We have quoted extensively and done our best to balance positive and negative responses.

When were you first concerned about your child?

The ages in our survey range from 12 months to 3 years. In the AFASIC survey 95 per cent of parents recognised that their child was having a difficulty by the age of four years and more than 50 per cent by the age of two. In one or two cases parents were clearly concerned about a number of aspects of their child's development before they were concerned about speech and language. In others, no concerns were expressed about any other skills.

What did you do about it?

The first point of call for most parents was their local health clinic often to see their clinic doctor, health visitor or general practitioner (GP). Sometimes this was in the context of a routine developmental check. At other times parents specifically sought help.

What sort of response did you get?

For some parents the first port of call was their local speech and language therapist. For many others the first person with whom parents had contact was their family doctor or health visitor. In some cases the doctor or health visitor assumed that hearing was the problem and referred the child on for a hearing test. One parent reported that grommets were fitted even though the hearing was adequate. Some parents felt that their concerns did not receive appropriate consideration. One spoke of 'being treated as a fussing new mum'. Clearly some parents have experienced difficulties getting their message across.

> After they [the doctor] had monitored the situation he was eventually referred to speech therapy at the age of three and a half years.

> We felt that we were floundering around for over a year waiting to see someone, not sure we were seeing the right person and being told to wait until he was older to see if there was a problem.

The question was raised as to how you get an assessment, particularly if your GP is not sympathetic. Obviously you need to start by being sure about your observations of your child. One parent commented in this context:

> Many early developmental signs are missed because people think that the child will grow out of them. My wife and I found it useful to keep a diary which helped identify problems and made it easier to explain them to others.

Some children were referred at a relatively early stage to an educational psychologist.

> We took her to a paediatrician who agreed she was not firing on all cylinders and recommended taking her to an educational psychologist.

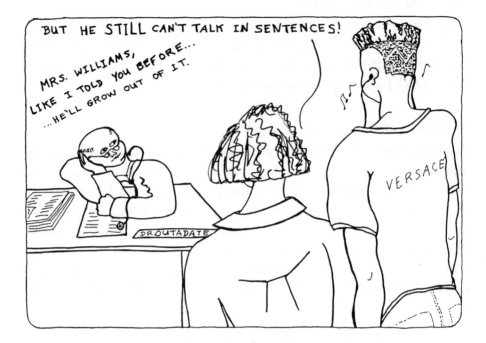

Figure 1

What experience did you have of specific professionals?

A number of parents were very pleased with the way the professionals treated their children. Comments such as:

> The help and assistance we have received has been first class and consistent throughout.

Others reported a much more variable response, treated sympathetically by some and less so by others. One parent reported:

> X was incredibly rude and decided that because we did not live in a tower block and my husband was not on the dole or spending 90 per cent of his time in the pub that we did not need any help and said so at our first meeting.

Another said:

> I found X to have no real experience of language difficulties and because of his personality considered that, because he knew nothing about it, the situation did not exist. I found him an

inexperienced, self-opinionated individual, an 'expert' who did not wish to consider anything other than what he had learned to date.

X was confused about his condition. With one exception, I found her unhelpful and rigid in her thinking. She was unable to consider or accommodate anything but the norm.

What sort of contact have you had with the speech and language therapy service? What did they say about your child and what did they do about it?

The response to the speech and language therapist was generally very favourably reported, although reservations were occasionally expressed about the time spent on waiting lists. Some parents made particular reference to specific therapists who had worked with their child. Others referred to a particular service. One parent wrote:

It was the speech therapists who explained to me what was wrong with my son; his likely prognosis; what course of action was open to me and what help I could expect from the local authority.

We asked parents whether they had been made aware of the options that were available to them for their child. Many said that they only found out what was available at a later date.

Did you feel that the professionals concerned were in agreement about what was needed for your child?

Most of our respondents reported that the professionals agreed with one another regarding their child's needs, although for some there had clearly been less consensus. One said:

If you get too many opinions it gets confusing. If parents find a professional unhelpful they should be encouraged to get another opinion and should not be labelled difficult.

while another had an altogether less favourable reaction:

No, I felt confusion and apathy from the professionals – and not much action.

Were you satisfied with the service that you received? If not, why not?

The majority of parents were clearly satisfied with the service that they received. One parent expressed anxiety about the early treatment in the following way:

> It felt that we spent a long time feeling hopeless while waiting for a course which you never get to go on. When he was offered group speech therapy others did not turn up and there were no groups. We were then offered another group after waiting and ringing constantly to see when we would be on the course.

Others have a more general complaint:

> Most of the people we have seen have either not taken us seriously or have got the situation completely wrong.

What sort of information would you have liked to receive?

One parent clearly expressed her satisfaction:

> I got all the information I needed and am very pleased with the service.

Some felt that they could have benefited from more information and help. Here are some examples:

> When we started out I was amazingly ignorant about language development. Our older boy had picked it all up so quickly that we had not given it a second thought. We have learned a great deal over the years. I only wish the information which we have picked up from all over the place had been available to us earlier on.

> [We would have liked to know] everything that could have helped our son with his speech at an early age.

> I would have liked to know what to expect, how slow the process is and, of course, we would have liked more therapy courses for the children. The group treatment that we received was more for parents than children but it helped us a great deal. We badly needed to talk to other parents.

> [We would have liked] information on other facilities and other therapies.

I would have liked clearly written reports not just those produced for the medical records. They need to be in language that can be easily understood.

Of course, it is often easier to think what you would have wanted after the event. One parent said very frankly:

Not knowing what was going on I did not know what to expect.

What sort of provision/treatment would you have liked to receive?

Where they had insight into this issue parents usually referred to the amount of help available:

Just more – what we received was great once we got it, although even Paul found it a bit too repetitive and we could see that it was a little easy at times.

Guaranteed provision within the borough for children with special needs. Good provision is short and one is made to fight and push all the way to make sure that your child gets a fair chance of receiving some of that provision.

I would like to have seen more awareness of speech and language disorders amongst GPs and health visitors.

At one stage in our son's development he was put in a special school where the teacher did not understand why he was unable to understand instructions. We then pressed for more refined education which would be targeted to his needs. He now attends a school for children with speech and language disorders and is making progress.

Other members of the family need to be educated about the child's disability. We have found that too often our son is thought of as retarded rather than have specific areas of language difficulty.

And with regard to the older child:

It would also be helpful for parents of older children to know what provision can be made beyond school leaving age and if local authorities have any obligation towards children who need to have their education extended. My own son, now aged 14, is unlikely to be ready to take up employment or to be fully socialised by the age of 16.

How involved were you with the therapy?

All the parents that we asked were very involved with therapy. Often this meant simply carrying out exercises that were set. In some cases it was rather more demanding of the parents.

> The therapy included me a lot. We were constantly videoed which I hated but I could see why it was done and, in the end, it was a very useful tool indeed. I turned up to all the sessions except for one when I was in hospital giving birth to his baby sister and I rang to cancel while in labour three hours before the delivery.

Would you have preferred to have had more involvement? If so, of what kind?

Most of the parents that we spoke to were happy with their level of involvement. In one case a parent of a child who had subsequently gone to a language unit expressed the wish that she had been more involved in the work of the unit. In other words, while it is relatively easy for parents to be involved when the children are attending clinic sessions, they may become more distanced from the process once their child is offered a 'placement'. Parents have to be aware that in pushing for an educational placement for their child, they may have to work harder to be included when they achieve what they have been pushing for.

> I believe parents and professionals should work together hand in hand to get the best out of the child. I believe that this has been the case in my situation.

One parent expressed concern about the involvement of other parents:

> I just wish that others were as committed as us. Unless parents were made to sign a contract they let the others down. I must add that I am very fortunate as I have not had to take time off work and had someone to look after my other child. This must be a big problem for others and transport could be a problem for some.

It is often difficult for parents to be precise about what, if any, improvement there might have been. One parent commented:

> It would have been helpful to know what he needed to learn at home and if so what books he could have read.

For others there is a growing awareness about the need for their own involvement:

> Initially I felt that the "experts" were in control and knew what they were doing. So at that time, no. However, in view of what I now know, yes, we should have been much more actively involved.

What sort of diagnosis did your child receive and has it changed over time? Did the diagnosis that you received match up to what you thought was wrong with your child?

The AFASIC survey showed that the majority of children were diagnosed some time after being identified. For a final diagnosis, a third of parents relied on the diagnosis made by the speech and language therapist. Some parents had a clear understanding that a diagnosis may change over time:

> John was diagnosed as having a language delay. This is now seen as more of a language disorder.

> We were told that Kassim had a language impairment. We thought that he was slow with his speech because he was bright in every other way.

> Clare showed a marked language disorder which has improved due to the help that she has received, but her language is still not what it should be for her age.

> He just needed speech therapy when he was under five and we agreed with that at the time, but as he got older it appeared that he needed more help.

> He is language disordered with both gross and fine motor problems.

> After having our son diagnosed 'autistic', it has now been changed to 'language disability'. When I told the headteacher of the autistic school that our son had attended, that there was a confusion as to whether he was autistic or not, her reply was that 'autism' was just a label.

Labels and their application was a salient feature of the discussion of all parents.

Can you describe how you felt when you were given the diagnosis and what impact did it have on your family life?

For some parents this seemed to be a difficult question because it meant little:

> We were fine. It was what he needed that was more important.

> Very little since we knew that there was something wrong and putting a name to it did not make a difference.

> We were pleased that Clare's problems could and would be improved by the special educational services that she was offered.

> Jim's diagnosis did not have any big impact on our family because we all feel that with time his speech will be just as normal as anyone else's. We think he is just a bit slow.

For other parents it is not so easy to handle:

> I felt devastated at first because no one wants to have a child who is not 100 per cent healthy. At first I blamed myself, e.g. I must have done something wrong when I was carrying him; was it his diet?; was it his childminder?; was it because I went to work?; was it something I should have picked up from the outset? Otherwise we have always had a very happy family life and his problem has made no difference whatsoever.

> Although he has made good progress with his speech therapy, the gap between him and his peers has widened. His problems have changed as he has got older and he needs constant re-assessment. We have wondered about many diagnoses – e.g. dyspraxia – as each new name is thrown at us.

> We have at times been almost desperate to know what is wrong – why? and whose fault is it? We were devastated when they suggested possible cerebral insult. We thought that the doctors thought that we had done something to him ourselves. We recognise now that it is just a term that is used, but it worried us very much at the time.

The impact of following an incorrect path and subsequent inactivity has been very frustrating. The apathy and inactivity of others has caused me to be very angry.

Do you feel that the implications were sufficiently well explained?

Again we had a divergence of opinion here. Some parents were very happy:

Yes, very well. I was always kept very well informed and had the opportunity to talk about my son at all times.

Others less so:

Not really – but they say we will never know why – which is very hard to live with as there is a lot of blame from both sides of our families. Steven has not been 'pigeon holed', which is good, but this means that we cannot find other parents with similar children who we can talk to.

Were you offered information regarding other agencies which might be useful to you?

A few parents had received no assistance of this kind, despite the fact that it is a duty for health professionals to provide this kind of information. Of the others, a number reported that they had been put in touch with the Association For All Speech Impaired Children and that the experience had been very helpful. Obviously expectations of such organisations are high and not always met. One parent expressed concern that she was sent:

Nothing but a load of rubbish about meetings and how much money they now have. What we needed was to be put in touch with other frustrated parents.

One parent referred to being put in touch with the Dyspraxia Trust, but:

I ended up telling the other two people there about how to statement their children – so that was a lost cause.

However, as we shall see in Chapter 9, these organisations have a great many enquiries and provide an invaluable information service and rallying point for scores of parents and professionals.

Do you feel that any attention was paid to what you said?

Most responded favourably to this and had no complaints. One, however, replied:

> I think that we, as parents, were unfortunately treated like the children. I know it was not meant, but sometimes we were spoken to in a very condescending manner.

Another indicated that it was not until they made a stand that they were taken seriously:

> Not until January when I prepared a very factual written report clearly stating how angry and frustrated I was and clearly showing that David's education was not helping him at all.

From a number of parents there was a feeling that they were seen as a nuisance because they had been complaining so much:

> I would like to see my LEA more receptive to parents who, in the view of the LEA, 'step out of line' on behalf of their children.

Can you describe your child's progress?

For parents wanting to know about the services and what is available, one of the first questions is always how much progress children can be expected to make. Some parents are very emphatic about the changes:

> Progress has been very good, she has made a lot of progress.

> He has made a lot of progress since he started at the language unit and he is reading much more fluently than he was.

> George has progressed enormously. Each day his speech seems to improve.

> John has made great progress albeit sometimes slower than others. He has now started in the language unit and enjoys it very much.

For others it has been more of a struggle:

> He can now string three or four words together and we can communicate reasonably well sometimes. He still says a load of nonsense and baby language/sounds. He still dribbles, but not as often as before. His fine motor skills are a bit better now, but his gross motor problems are still very apparent.

What do you think has most helped him/her over the years?

Parents seem to have a pretty clear idea of what has most helped their child and for most the praise went to the specialised unit in which the child had been placed.

> Intensive group therapy sessions every day for nine weeks. I wish there had been more of them.

> The early childhood language unit and the assistance given to him by his class teacher and the headteacher at school.

> Having her special needs met by being in a language class and having more individual attention than she would have received in a mainstream school.

> When he first went into the language unit, that helped him more than having [weekly] speech therapy.

For others, the parents' role was seen as more important.

> Parental tenacity and our refusal to give up have been most important for us. We should add that the stress and strain that has resulted has, at times, caused family upsets.

What help would you have liked most that you did not receive?

A number of parents replied 'none' to this question. However, some had suggestions, often relating to the amount of speech and language therapy services that they received. Many were of a quite general nature:

> Not enough speech therapy courses offered, but great when received. I feel very sorry for the parents that are less able to understand that unless you know who to keep ringing and pushing they will not get the help that their children need.

For others the need seems to have been broader:

> Better coordination of services and more centralised information.

> He would have been helped by mixing more with people of different ages. It has always been a struggle trying to get him involved with different activities.

> The role of social workers in helping families with disabled children should be covered.

What advice would you give to anyone whose child has recently been identified as being language impaired?

All parents felt that they had something to say to other parents:

> See as many specialists and find out as much as you can.

> Once your child is ready to be in a group, make contact with the other parents and compare notes. You will then realise that they also have children with not only language problems, but bad behaviour, sleepless nights and many other similar experiences. It can be a time when you feel very much on your own but you only have to see the long waiting lists [for speech and language therapy] to know that you are not. Don't bury your head in the sand and I'm afraid that you will have to battle constantly for places and to get the statement sorted out. But the more you know, however upsetting it may seem, the more it will pay rewards later.

> I would tell them to know their own child, listen to what the professionals have to say but make their own choices. Talk with the child as much as you can and get them to keep a conversation going with you about all sorts of things.

> Seek every help through every channel that you find and persist until you get what you want.

> Take your child to a speech therapist as early as possible. Once you are in the system things move onwards and you can find out what else is on offer for your child.

> Seek professionals' help; gather together as much information as you can on your child's impairment and join a support group.

For some, the advice was more specific:

> I would stress the importance of getting the statement right, so that it clearly states the children's needs and is not written in such an ambiguous way that it can be interpreted to suit local authority resources. Not checking the statement carefully was an error that we made and it seemed almost impossible to correct at a later stage. AFASIC gave us advice later, on what should appear on the statement.

Summary

It is important to recognise that although we spoke to a number of parents, it is never possible to say that the views expressed are representative of all parents. Clearly there will be some who would not agree with what has been expressed here. Services will vary depending upon where you live in the country, and personal experiences of professionals is bound to differ considerably.

Similarly, we know that these children are so different from one another that it is often very difficult to group them at all. They have their own individual strengths and weaknesses. Consequently, it is unlikely that your child or your circumstances will be reflected exactly in the comments made above. Your level of concern and your experience of 'the system', together with your son or daughter's age and pattern of abilities, will determine which are relevant to your circumstances.

If we were to summarise the findings above, most parents seem to have expressed frustration with the system somewhere or other. But as they come to know their child's strengths and weaknesses and once they come to form relationships with the professionals involved, they are, for the most part, very satisfied with the help that they have received once they get it. Clearly determination is an essential ingredient for any parent trying to find help for their child.

A strong feeling emerged that parents wanted more information about language and language difficulties and how the system could help them and their child. It was in response to this that we decided to produce this book. In the final analysis, the point that we want to make to you as parents, and indeed to the professionals who you encounter, is that a service that does not take the parents' views into consideration at every step of the process of identification and treatment, can never really be called a service.

CHAPTER 2

Getting Started
The Development of Speech and Language

Katey is eight weeks old. She knows her mother and her father by their voice and their faces and indicates her interest in them relative to sounds that she hears. Much of the time she is busy kicking but she will still to sounds of noisy toys on her cot. She makes a great many little involuntary sounds and both her mother and her father make great play of interpreting what she means, exaggerating the intonation in their voices as they do so.

How does it all start?

It is sometimes thought that children do not start communicating until they learn to speak. But if we look at a baby closely, it is clear that she[1] is trying to make contact with those around within days of being born. At first it may be a cry or fleeting eye contact and it is difficult to be sure what the child was intending to communicate. But watch her parents. They will be interpreting what she is meaning to say from the word go. Most parents actively try to include the baby by reading in what she is meaning. Parents often joke about whether the baby's grimace is a smile or due to wind. The important point is that we want to call it a smile even if it is not.

We know that children are tuned into sound from the very beginning and quickly learn to locate familiar voices and distinguish them from those

---

1   Throughout the text we will be using 'she' as the neutral term to refer to children. We shall be using 'he' to refer to children with speech or language impairments.

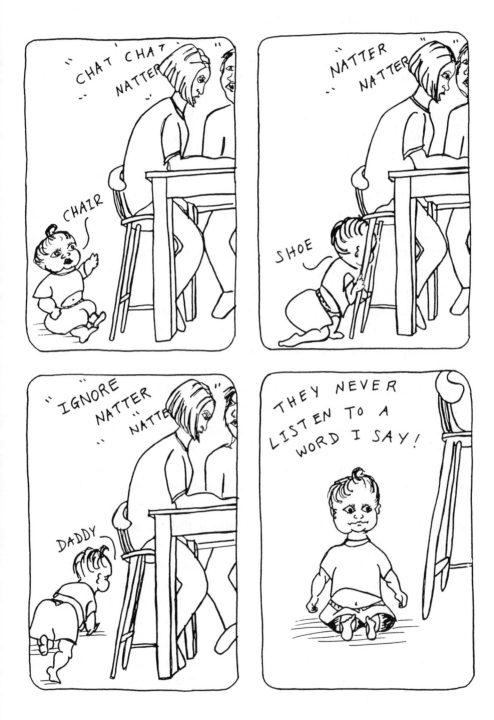

Figure 2

that are less familiar. Similarly, babies are excited by more pronounced tones in the voices of the adults around them. Many people have argued that babies are pre-programmed to communicate and the speed with which they seem to acquire these skills makes it very hard to disagree.

The first year is marked by an increase in the child's conscious control. Gradually she begins to hold objects and then manipulate them. Soon this control is extended to the sounds that she makes. She begins to play with sounds and the sounds reflect the child's feelings. She coos when she is happy and screams when not given the right sort of attention. Again the parent has to use informed guess work to establish what is the right sort of attention. This is important because it requires the parent to understand what the child is trying to say and then meet the need in question. Although it is clearly true that humans are programmed to communicate, they only really do so if they have something to communicate about and they know that their message will be listened to and understood.

Some have described this early interaction as a dance, with parent and child as partners. Both participants learn the steps that they need to communicate effectively. Initially the adult takes the lead and provides 'scaffolding' for the child to continue, but gradually the child begins to take initiatives, to start off interaction for herself. Research suggests that the rhythms associated with this dance are extremely predictable and are the same for a wide range of different cultures. Indeed it has even been suggested that the beat speeds up from adagio to andante and to moderato in the first six to nine months. As the child begins to initiate, she learns that a certain noise or facial expression is appropriate in a given situation and she begins to exploit this almost as if she is telling an old familiar joke. The parent then recognises and reinforces this and the dance continues. We see the parent emphasising the intonation with facial expression, exaggerating the intended meaning.

Objects, too, come to play an ever-increasing role in the interaction. As the child develops conscious control over her movements, she reaches for interesting objects and brings them to her mouth. She manipulates them with increasing skill and gradually learns that objects have specific predictable functions. Even relatively young children know that a comb goes to the head or a telephone head set to the ear. Thus the child's skills come together, so that by the end of the first year she has all the necessary capacities to start using language to communicate.

The importance of that first year cannot be overestimated. We could argue that it is here that the first conversations develop and it is the desire to converse with others which drives the child forward in her acquisition of communication skills as she gets older. If she enjoys chatting with her mother, that is all the more reason to try it out on others. And the more practice you receive, the more skillful you will become. In recent years there has been increasing interest in these conversational skills and it is now widely recognised that although these skills continue to develop throughout the school years, they start from the word 'go'!

Listening

Before children learn to speak, they have to learn to listen. In some cases, children are at a considerable disadvantage because they have hearing losses. We will be discussing these further in Chapter 6, but for the moment it is important that we know how well a child is hearing. Parents usually notice when children have marked difficulties, but find it hard to distinguish children with milder problems from those who simply do not want to do what they are asked.

As they develop an interest in tuning in to others, children with normal hearing begin to make sense of what is said around them. We are not quite sure how much they take from the language that they hear around them in the first year, although recent studies suggest that children can distinguish between verbs and nouns by about ten months. They clearly process the link between the words that they hear and the context in which those words are said. Indeed one of the first communicative events strictly under the control of the child emerges around the tenth month when they point to an object, drawing it to the attention of a familiar adult. In other words they are saying 'I know it's there and I know that you know it too'. The delight on the child's face and the insistence in their voice shows us how important this communication is. They would not be able to do this unless they had first seen adults doing the same for them.

Initially, children become preoccupied with the objects which interest them. Anyone who tries to distract them from their purpose is in for a rude awakening. But gradually they learn that you can focus on something for a while, leave it for something else or to listen to someone speaking and then come back to the object. By two or three years of age children will stop playing with a toy to listen and then go back to it. By four they are often able to integrate what is said to them without leaving the toy at all. They can continue playing while taking in what is said to them.

Listening is one of the most important of all the skills that children need if they are to learn from their environment.

Verbal comprehension

Although children make use of all sorts of information to make sense of the world (eye contact, posture, facial expression etc), for them to make sense of language it must be meaningful to them. They must be able to extract information which they can understand from what they hear. It is little wonder that children do not listen if they are not able to understand what is said to them and if they don't listen then understanding doesn't develop. But what do we mean by verbal comprehension?

We need to draw a distinction between what children understand simply by being familiar with the context in which it is said and what they are able to understand purely from the words that they hear. Parents often say of young children that they understand everything that is said to them. In many cases this is probably unlikely. Rather, the children make use of the context and of all the communicative information that they have already acquired to guess what has been said. Perhaps they hear a single word and anticipate the meaning of a sentence. Perhaps they see an eye gaze or a finger point or hear an intonation pattern in the parent's speech that leads them to the correct response. Take, for example, a situation in which a mother asks her two-and-a-half-year-old to 'go and find your coat behind the door in the kitchen'. If the coat is routinely kept there, the single word 'coat' is probably all she needs to respond correctly. And even this may be redundant if he has seen his mother put on her hat, coat and gloves, an obvious signal that she is going out.

As we shall see in the next chapter, speech and language therapists often restrict use of the term 'verbal comprehension' to the type of exercise in which the child has to choose between a carefully controlled number of items. Thus the child will be shown a doll, a teddy bear, a cup and a spoon. She will first be asked to point to the individual items. Then she will be asked to give the spoon to dolly. If the child can identify the objects, but not make sense of the associations, he is said to be at a 'one-word level' of verbal comprehension. If he is able to make the connections necessary to carry out this type of request he is at a 'two-word level' and so on. By the age of three most children can process specific requests with three or four ideas in them. These ideas are sometimes called 'information-carrying words', to distinguish them from the other words in the sentence which may be less important. These terms will be discussed at greater length in Chapters 5 and 8.

It is important to recognise that comprehension is made up of a number of skills. The most obvious of these is memory. A child who finds it difficult to remember will struggle in learning words and in doing so will often take longer to understand requests that are made. Vocabulary is similarly important. Children build up a substantial understanding of words within the first two or three years so that they can interpret any new word which they hear as having a given meaning and slot it into what they already know. Thus, if the child already has a word for mouse, cat, dog and rabbit and then hears the word 'gerbil' in the context of a small furry animal, it will be relatively simple to put this new word along side the others and classify them together. If he does not already have some sort of category for small furry animals, it will be that much more difficult to retain the new word. This problem becomes more acute as the child gets older. If a child has difficulty acquiring new words, then it will be more difficult to process requests and extract information from what he hears around him. By two or three years of age children are able to match new words that they hear to what they already know at considerable speed. It is important that this is an active process in which the child engages. Some people maintain that language can be taught. However, it is virtually impossible to teach children new words unless they are relevant to the child's experience.

As the child moves into nursery and on to school she must learn not only that words have meaning in themselves and that they can be arranged in such a way that 'the dog chased the cat' and the 'cat chased the dog' do not mean the same thing, but she must also know that speakers can use words in different ways to change meaning. They must learn that a teacher who says 'who's a busy little girl?' with a certain intonation pattern is being sarcastic and does not expect the answer 'me'. She must learn that words like 'stand' often refer to your physical posture, but may also relate to your tolerance level. 'I can't stand this mess' will mean little to the child who retains only the most literal interpretation of the word 'stand'. Similarly, children at this age are learning to joke with language, jokes which they can share with their peers. A child who does not have a good understanding of the vocabulary and grammar of language will struggle in interpreting these more complex uses of language.

Speech

When they refer to communication most people think of speech. This is, of course, the most obvious aspect of it, although there are all sorts of skills underpinning communication which are not 'speech' as such. Speech concerns the mechanical production of recognisable sounds and involves an extremely complex interaction between breath control, coordination of the lips, tongue and palate, and interpretation of the signals coming from the brain. Given that these are probably the most complex skills we will ever learn, it is no wonder that in the first few years so many children struggle with aspects of it. Of course, some children excel in this area just as some are good at climbing or sorting shapes.

As we shall see in the next chapter, a distinction is often drawn between a number of different aspects of speech, notably **articulation, voice, phonology** and the **coordination of speech. Articulation** represents the individual's physical capacity to produce sounds and depends on the structures in the mouth (tongue, palate, teeth etc) and the way in which the child is able to use them. A child with a cleft palate is likely to have air escaping through the nose. A child with a very large tongue may well have difficulties producing certain sounds. In both cases the child's articulation will be affected. By contrast, a child who has poor use of the vocal folds may strain her **voice** so that it becomes hoarse. This condition is relatively uncommon in young children but it does show that it is possible for the child's voice quality to be affected. More commonly children have difficulty in getting the right volume for their speech. It is common for children who have language and speech difficulties to be reported by their parents to whisper or shout inappropriately.

Every language includes a different **phonological system** or set of phonological sounds, some of which will overlap with those in other languages and some will not. This becomes all too apparent when we try to pronounce the words of a language with which we are unfamiliar. Inevitably we interpret the sounds of that language in terms of those in our own. We know that from birth children become sensitised to the sounds of their own language and subsequently learn to predict where the boundaries between words come – effectively where words start and stop. They are then likely to become confused when first exposed to another language. As the child then comes to produce her own words, the sounds come to correspond to those of the first language. It is worth noting here that children exposed to more than one language simultaneously in the first few years of life soon learn to discriminate the sounds of both languages perfectly adequately. It is generally understood that children come to acquire new sounds by comparing those that they do know with those with which they are unfamiliar. Within a given language children then come to acquire new sounds in a very predictable way. They generally start with the *vowels* (a, e, i, o, u), but rapidly acquire *plosives*, especially those produced at the front of the mouth (p/b, t/d). Gradually they come to produce sounds produced at the back of the mouth (k/g). Often the speech of very young children is characterised by a use of this range of sounds.

However, without the *fricatives* (f, sh, s, v, th), it will be very difficult for a listener to decipher what has been said. These have usually started to emerge by the age of two years or so, although children may not have mastered the coordination of their production of the sounds 's' and 'th' until they are five or so. More subtle sound changes have still to be made. The *affricates* ('ch' as in 'change' and 'j' as in 'John') come in by most children's fourth birthday although many continue to make slight confusions with these and with groups of sounds such as the *liquids* (l, r) and the *glides* (w, y). The important point to remember is not that children necessarily have to have learned specific sounds by specific ages, but that they are making progress and their ability to make themselves understood is keeping up with what they are trying to say.

Finally, we turn to the **coordination of speech**. This refers to the individual's capacity to coordinate their muscles effectively. It is all very well having the structures of the mouth functioning well, and a good understanding of the sounds which need to be made to produce a given word, but if the brain cannot tell the tongue and lips what to say, the speech sounds are likely to become confused. The term sometimes used for this coordination is **praxis** and children who experience a difficulty acquiring these skills are sometimes called **dyspraxic**. These and other diagnostic terms will be discussed further in Chapter 5. Praxis suggests the concept of 'practice' and indeed speech production relies on the child developing ways of producing sounds in an automatic fashion. It is as if the child needs to build up a **motor programme** for a given sound or sequence of sounds. This programme is then activated at the appropriate moment. The more the child practises, the more likely these sound sequences are to become automatic.

From the earliest sounds that the child makes, these sound sequences are being exercised and as phonological skills develop, so too do those of coordination. Indeed it is often very difficult to disentangle the two. Unfortunately there is still a great deal which we need to find out about praxis. Why is it that some children seem to be so coordinated from the start, while others struggle to lay down the appropriate motor patterns? We do not know what is 'enough' practice to allow the child to produce sounds appropriately. It is not uncommon for any young children to trip up as they speak. For many this is likely to be a sign of **normal non-fluency** associated with the process of acquiring the automatic process of language. Of course, for some, it is an indication of later difficulties with fluency and such behaviour should never be ignored.

What other skills are involved?

Language does not develop in a vacuum but as a function of a number of different skills and abilities and these must be taken into consideration if we are to understand language development.

Hearing

When children are born, their hearing is as good as it will ever be. Of course they do not often know what they are listening to, but they have the capacity to hear what is going on around them. They can hear and distinguish familiar voices and it is not long before they can recognise words. As their own language skills develop, they need to be able to keep up with conversation. This tests their hearing to the utmost. As we shall see in the next chapter there are children who have hearing difficulties at birth and need help tuning into those early sounds. Similarly there are children whose hearing is fine at birth but deteriorates because their middle ear has become blocked after colds or ear infections. It is of paramount importance that difficulties that the child is experiencing because of hearing loss are identified as soon as possible. The longer she experiences a reduction of what she hears, the greater the likelihood that this may interfere with her language. Hearing losses of one sort or another are probably the simplest explanations for subsequent speech and language difficulties for many children. Of course, as we shall see, many children with difficulties in their communication skills do not have difficulties hearing. However, it must never be overlooked.

Memory

Conventionally, memory is separated out into long-term and short-term memory. A child must be able to hold what she hears for long enough to make sense of it, to store the information alongside the other bits of information related to the subject. She must also be able to keep it in that store so that she can come back and use it at another point in time. It is not useful to learn a word in the short-term and lose it later on. To a certain extent, of course, we all do this. We are aware that we know a word, but we cannot seem to get at it. In such cases it would probably be more accurate to say that we have not actually lost the word but are simply experiencing a difficulty retrieving it. We sometimes speak of this as being on the 'tip of the tongue' and we may be able to develop strategies which allow us access to the word that we are looking for. If this happens too often it can severely interfere with our communication.

Too little is known about the relationship between memory and language to be clear how they interact. Certainly children with better language skills seem to have better short-term memories. This is understandable because it is just these children who have a wider store of words with which to cross reference what they know. When they hear the word 'bench' in context they can quickly associate it with all the other words that they know for objects that they sit on. A child who does not have these other words may have difficulty making the appropriate associations when the word is heard and this may make it very difficult to store it effectively.

Symbolic skills

When we learn that the word 'dog' refers to a furry animal with four legs that barks, we are learning about a symbolic relationship. The word 'dog' only comes to mean what it does because we accept the relationship between the word and the object. After all, if we started calling dogs something else it would be rather confusing for those around us. The need to understand the symbolic nature of this relationship is reflected in the relationship between toys and the real world. Even very small children know that a doll is a doll and not a real person. Yet that does not stop them imbuing the doll with all sorts of human characteristics.

For many children, this type of **symbolic play** is closely related to their overall language development. Those with well-advanced symbolic play are often those with good language development. Although this is not always the case, the reverse does seem to be true. Those who have difficulty playing creatively with toys often have difficulty in manipulating language. It is unclear exactly what the relationship between the two is. Clearly there are children who manage to learn language perfectly well without being particularly skilled in this area. Indeed in some cultures relatively little attention is given to the type of activity which would be called play in the West. Yet we do not know that the children's language development in such cases is at all adversely affected. It seems probable that the type of symbolic play setting to which we are referring – dolls' tea parties and the like – offers a great many opportunities for children to develop their social language and that those who do customarily engage in such activities with adults and others who are able to shape and model language for them, do end up with more advanced language skills.

Non-verbal skills

There is also a host of other skills which the child employs to make sense of her world. Some, like the ability to recall and relate sequences, are clearly associated with language. Others such as hand and eye coordination are less obviously associated. These abilities are often loosely referred to as cognitive skills. Although these skills may contribute to the child's language development, the question arises as to whether they are necessary for it to proceed. There remains much discussion as to whether language skills are somehow different from those needed for other aspects of the child's development. We do know that children have quite different strengths and weaknesses and that some may be poor in their use of language, while good in other areas and vice versa (see Chapter 4 for a further discussion). It is, however, probable that children who have a wide range of learning difficulties relative to their peers, will also have difficulties with their language.

The development of grammar

We have already looked at the way in which speech develops over the pre-school period but the same is, of course, true of other parts of the language system. For example, if we look at the development of grammar, we see the shift in the second year from single words to short phrases. Initially children produce nouns and then verbs, but gradually they begin to expand them into phrases and clauses. Thus 'juice' for the 18-month-old becomes 'drink juice' by two, 'daddy drink juice' or 'no drink juice' by two and a half, 'daddy's drinking juice in a cup' by three and 'daddy's drinking juice and I'm eating dinner' by three and a half. Children continue to elaborate by using relative clauses 'the dinner, *that I'm eating,* is yummy' and passive constructions 'the dinner was eaten by the dog' and by four or five years of age they are well on their way to achieving most of the adult grammatical system. Vocabulary develops apace and children practise how to use new words by slotting them into existing constructions and monitoring the response of experienced users of the language. We often notice the cute things that children say, 'I go-ded to the shops', but what is remarkable is not that they make these errors but that they make comparatively few of them.

Alongside the development of grammar comes an ever-increasing elaboration of the child's capacity to classify the world – their *semantic system.* Whereas the two-year-old may over extend the meaning of 'dog' to mean all sorts of furry animals the five-year-old has become very precise in her use of words. She knows which words refer to animals and which do not. She knows about what many of them eat and something about their habitat. She may know the difference between mammals, birds and fish, and even why they are different. As she is exposed to new words for animals she is able to infer which category they should be put into according to their attributes (wings, eggs etc). Similarly she knows that there are different forms of verbs – transitive (those that take objects) and intransitive (those that do not). Although she will not know the terms, she understands about different structures.

The use of language

Perhaps most remarkable of all, by five years, she has learned how to communicate effectively with her peers. She is able to negotiate for what she wants, to ask for something in a certain way in the knowledge that she is more likely to receive it. She is aware of how others feel about the world and is able to take this into consideration. She knows how to tell lies and, of course, that she should not. She knows something about telling jokes and the function that this serves. She is coming to learn about the difference between what adults say in terms of the words and phrases that they use and what they actually mean when they use these constructions. In other words, the five-year-old is moving beyond simply learning language to learning about the way that it works in the culture in which she is growing up.

It is important to bear in mind that there are numerous subtleties in the way in which language is used in different cultures and that a child may end up with knowledge specific to her own culture but find it difficult to extend this to others with whom she comes into contact. We see this especially acutely in the school playground where children have to negotiate their values with their peers. In other words, the child's language development is not simply a matter of learning words and grammar: it is the way that these parts are put together to make sense to other people that is especially important. For example, the child (aged six) in the following sequence clearly has gone beyond the grammar of her mother's sentence in constructing her response.

MOTHER: 'Joanne will you go to the shops for me?'

JOANNE: 'I'm not allowed in the off licence.'

Instead, she has used her knowledge of her own experience to interpret what her mother had intended. We do this all the time, but it is not something that it is possible to assess in any formal sense because it is so particular to the relationship between the speaker and listener.

Moving into school

The child's language skills are inevitably linked to her capacity to read and write. Just as the baby learns how to chop up the sounds that she hears into recognisable words, so the young school-age child learns the link between the sounds that she hears and says, and the letters that go to make up the words that she first recognises and subsequently writes. Apart from learning how to reproduce the shapes of the letters when she writes them, she must learn that there are rules to be followed. In some languages the relationship between the sounds of the language and the letters used to represent them is fairly straightforward. The child then knows that whenever she encounters a letter it will always be said in the same way. In English, however, there are a great many irregularities which need to be learned by means of specific rules e.g. 'i' before 'e' except after 'c'. These irregularities are the result of a very complex cultural and linguistic history and they often prove an obstacle for children starting to read. Although, for many, the process of learning to associate language and reading appears effortless, it is important to recognise that it is a complex process requiring an integration of all that the child has learned about language up until that point. Having said that, most children have made tremendous progress in this area by the time they are seven. And once the world of books has been opened up to them, it is not long before they are able to teach themselves about their world, without necessarily waiting for a more experienced speaker to show them the way.

The level of information available to children has expanded dramatically in recent years. Whereas in the past children were restricted to the specific texts that they were able to find at school or at home, they are now in a position to benefit from a whole range of by-products of the information technology revolution. Computer literacy skills, which children now learn alongside their more conventional literacy skills, will allow children to access a world of information to which their parents had little access. The interactive CD Rom, for example, will soon be common place in the school and the home. For those who are able to use them there is no end of potential, not only for information, but also for the child's ability to teach herself. There is a common fear that the burst in information technology will lead to a world of unsocial computer boffins! In other words, the children's computer skills will have been trained up at the expense of their social skills – in effect at the expense of their capacity to use language, to infer the intended meaning of the person with whom they are conversing. While many of these concerns are probably unwarranted there is a genuine need to draw a distinction between the type of knowledge available through computing skills and the social communication skills which can only arise through interaction with others.

The introduction of the National Curriculum in the UK has had many implications for the way in which language is assessed in all state schools. Indeed most subjects are assessed through the medium of language and are, therefore, in some way a function of the child's linguistic skills. While it is probably unlikely that a child with good language skills who does not have an aptitude or an inclination for science will excel in this area, the reverse is probably true. Children who struggle with language are in great danger of being judged in all subjects on the basis of their language and not the subject in question. Thus a child who is quite able in technological subjects may be unable to express that ability through language and may therefore be assumed to be less able than she really is.

Although the journey takes place in a relatively short time period, a very long distance has been travelled between those first few words and the demands to which the child responds in school. There is a level which is within the reach of all but a very few children. How far they proceed once they have reached that basic level will depend on all sorts of factors, of which the child's inherent ability is only one. Parental expectations, the opportunities provided for the child and the child's motivation will all play their part in determining how far the child will progress as they go up the school. Language is one of the basic building blocks upon which they rely in the first instance. Without it, educational progress is likely to be effortful and slow.

Explanations

Parents sometimes ask what happens to the child's brain when she is developing language. This is, of course, not a very easy question to answer, because it is difficult to find out in any direct way. We cannot simply take the top off and have a look! We do know from work with adults that specific parts of the brain seem to be programmed to accept language. However, there has been some progress recently in our ability to scan the brain. By necessity, such studies as have been carried out have been small, because no one is keen to expose children to medical examinations that they do not need. Whereas it used to be assumed that children built up connections between different parts of the brain as they got older, it is now apparent that children are born with all the potential connections that they need and that as they develop, certain connections become more useful and remain, whereas others are not used and fade away. In other words, children lose connections between parts of the brain as they age. By the age of three most of the connections necessary for language development are in place. Nevertheless, there is evidence from children who have had brain injuries in the pre-school period that language can relocate to other parts of the brain with remarkable ease. We are still a long way from fully understanding this process.

Some have argued that children learn language only from what they hear. They argue that children are simply trained to use the appropriate linguistic forms much as they learn all sorts of other behaviours. Others suggest that there is an innate set of structures within the brain which are peculiar to humans and that a child will learn language with relatively little language around them. In other words, language learning is triggered by a complex interaction between brain development and the environment in which that development takes place, but that after this it proceeds much as a flower grows given water.

The reality is probably somewhere between these two positions. It is very unlikely that children could learn language as quickly as they do purely on the basis of what they hear. And anyway, if they did, they would probably repeat all the incomplete 'baby-like' things that adults say to them. Equally, it is clear that they are greatly influenced by what they hear for the quantity and quality of their subsequent language. It seems likely that children are born programmed actively to search out sense in what they perceive through their *auditory channel*, just as they try to make sense of patterns and come to discriminate familiar faces. While they are able to make progress on their own, they have much to gain from parents who provide them with opportunities to learn when they are ready to do so. If we go back to Katey, whom we first met at the beginning of this chapter, it is clear that she will learn more if we give her toys when she is ready for them. We know that there are times when she is busy and distracted and others when she stills and appears to listen. We know that she shows a preference for faces that she can see and hear at the same time. Without appropriate stimulation babies become fretful and listless. We know too that constant noise does little to help children make sense of their world.

Summary

The majority of children acquire language with considerable skill within a relatively short period of time. They follow similar patterns of development and by the time they reach school are skilful communicators. That so few children struggle with this process is indeed remarkable. Nevertheless, some children do find it difficult. They may do so for as many reasons as there are skills involved. In such cases parents often become concerned when the child is between the age of two and three years, and they look for help. In the UK the first stop is often the health visitor and thence the speech and language therapist and a full developmental assessment. The next chapter looks at the way that the speech and language therapist assesses such children and Chapter 4 describes the assessments made by other professionals whom parents are likely to encounter as they look to find out how they can best help their child.

CHAPTER 3

The Assessment

What Are Speech and Language Therapists Looking For?

This chapter is about what happens to your child once he has been identified as having speech or language difficulties. In particular we have concentrated on the role of the speech and language therapist in relation to your child. We talk about the type of information you will be asked for and try to explain what these assessments tell us, why they are important, and how they are carried out.

Referral

In the UK there is a national Child Health Surveillance programme which aims to offer developmental screening and thus early detection of a range of childhood difficulties including developmental delays, and speech and language difficulties. This screening is carried out in local clinics by health visitors, GP's and clinical medical officers (clinic doctors) and is likely to be the first point of contact for parents. The ages at which such screening takes place varies across the country but, for most children, the first prescribed screen specifically designed to pick up speech and language difficulties will occur at, or around, the time of the child's second birthday. There is some argument as to whether speech and language difficulties can be detected at an earlier age, but the range of 'normal language development' at this age is extremely wide and earlier screening produces considerable numbers of false–positive results, i.e. children who fail the screen and are referred for speech and language therapy, but who are subsequently found on assessment to have normal speech and language development.

Parents of children with speech and language difficulties are often aware by the time the child is two years, or even earlier, that their child is not developing language as other siblings or friends' children have done and may contact their GP or health visitor for advice at this time. Indeed parental judgement is one of the most important factors that professionals take into consideration when they assess a child. Children whose difficulties have gone undetected may have started nursery or school before receiving any professional help. In this instance the teacher may notice the child's difficulties and, following the stages of assessment laid down by the Department for Education in the 1994 Code of Practice (for schools) (see Chapters 7 and 10), will offer a period of assessment, review, setting and monitoring of individual teaching targets as part of the child's educational programme, and then refer, if necessary, to an outside agency such as a speech and language therapist for further advice.

The speech and language therapist

Speech and language therapists generally work for the NHS, have a degree in speech and language therapy and are qualified to work with both adults and children. They are usually based in community clinics and hospitals, and aim to provide services to them as well as mainstream and special schools or units. The therapist does not work in a vacuum, and is accountable to a service manager who will, in turn, have their own priorities as prescribed by the Trust Board, its purchasers, the regional health authority and ultimately current government initiatives and objectives. Waiting lists for first appointments and assessments by a speech and language therapist vary enormously and many services prioritise referrals according to a set of criteria amongst which one would expect to find:

1. The age of the child.

2. The level of (child/parent/school) concern.

3. The severity of the difficulty as described by the referring agent.

4. The impact of the difficulty on the child, family, school.

5. Whether one or more areas of difficulty are being experienced.

6. Length of time on the waiting list.

An appointment will usually be made for the child and his parents/carers to attend a local clinic. During this, and subsequent appointments for assessment, the therapist will want to gather a great deal of information from the parents, observe the child's means of communication, social interaction skills, non-verbal skills, attention, listening and play skills, and may carry out some formal speech and language assessments or tests. Throughout the information gathering, observation and formal assessment, the therapist will be looking to see if there *is* a problem, what sort of problem it is and how they can go about helping the child and his family.

What can parents expect during assessment?

Initially the therapist will take a case history. This will involve asking questions and gathering information from parents about various aspects of the child's development, together with discussion about what the parent perceives the child's difficulties to be and their possible causes. It is important that the therapist gains a picture of the whole child so that the difficulties he is experiencing acquiring speech and language can be seen as part of a pattern of strengths and weaknesses in his overall development. The therapist needs to identify the child's strengths as she will work through these to help the child.

Case history

A number of different areas of the child's development are covered in the case history. Commonly these may be separated into medical, social and cultural, developmental, communication and education history. We will now have a look at each in turn.

MEDICAL HISTORY

While collecting data on medical history, the therapist will be looking for 'significant' medical history and medical conditions which could have affected the child's speech and language or general development. For example, a child with an undetected and untreated hearing loss, a child who suffered anoxia (lack of oxygen) at birth, or a child who has been frequently hospitalised through illness or disability may have a medical cause for the presenting difficulty.

This information will form part of the body of knowledge required to make a diagnosis and plan future intervention for the child. Should the therapist feel that the child has a medical condition that has previously gone unrecognised, she will, after discussion with the family and other involved agencies (GP, health visitor, school), refer the child to the appropriate specialist agency, for example a child development centre.

SOCIAL AND CULTURAL HISTORY

Within different cultures and societies, and indeed individual families and schools, expectations of children's development and the rate at which they acquire new skills vary. It is important for the therapist to understand the expectations of the family and the cultural norms for each individual and his social group. Family language patterns and social environment will have an effect on speech and language development. There is some evidence to support the theory that some difficulties with speech and language are familial. There may also be a family history of such difficulties which have gone largely unnoticed as the presenting problems may, in the past, have been insufficiently pronounced to warrant referral.

Another issue which often proves to be very complex for speech and language therapists and other professionals, is the diagnosis of language impairments in the bilingual child. Although the majority of children exposed to more than one language become effortlessly bilingual, there are some who seem to struggle with the acquisition of language as a skill. These children often pose problems for parents and teachers trying to ascertain whether they really do have a difficulty. For example, it is often hard to decide whether they are simply slower in learning a particular language or whether they have similar difficulties in all the languages to which they are exposed. It is certainly more difficult for the therapist to make a **differential diagnosis** when more than one language is involved. The therapist will need a considerable amount of information about family language patterns and more importantly she will need to know how competent the family feel the child is and in which language. Where necessary, interpretors may be available to assist the family and the therapist, and assessment should be undertaken, as far as possible in the child's first or home language.

DEVELOPMENTAL HISTORY

In order to ascertain whether the child's speech and language difficulty is discrete, or part of a wider pattern of more general learning difficulties, the therapist will seek information about the child's development. There are developmental norms for motor – both gross and fine, cognitive, self-help, speech and language, and social communications skills, among others, and these norms provide an age range during which most children will acquire a given skill. For example, a child who has no known medical condition which would mitigate against 'normal' motor development, and has had the appropriate opportunities and encouragement to do so, would be expected to walk independently between 10 and 18 months.

A child's skills do not develop in isolation and when children's milestones (the age at which they acquire a skill) fall well outside the expected age range, it would be usual for clinicians to look for a reason for the delay. The impact and effect such a delay in acquiring one skill can have on the development of another varies. The therapist will need this information before she can give the family advice and provide the child with strategies with which to cope. Many of the skills a child needs to develop in order to be independent are related to one another. A limitation or delay in any one area of development may adversely affect another. For example, a child with delayed gross motor skills, who is less mobile and able to explore his environment, has more limited access to a range and variety of potentially stimulating learning experiences. This may in turn impede his development of language skills through lack of opportunity both to acquire different vocabulary, and to hear and use language in different meaningful contexts.

COMMUNICATION HISTORY

The therapist will also seek detailed information about the child's past and present communication skills. Information of this type will be considered not only within the parameters of 'developmental norms' for the development of speech and language, but also in consideration of the data gathered about the whole child's development to date. Time will be spent in discussion with parents, carers and teachers about the child's personality, behaviour, desire to communicate, and opportunities and experiences which have been presented to the child in order to facilitate the development of speech and language.

The variety of early communication histories is very wide indeed and it is often difficult to generalise from one child to another. Some children may have been quiet babies who rarely vocalised or babbled and did not attempt to imitate adult models of sounds and then single words; conversely some children have talked a good deal but the content of their language or *what* they say has been inappropriate and not meaningful in given contexts. It is important for the therapist to build a picture of the child's communication skills in a variety of contexts. Through discussion with significant people in the child's life (family, school etc), a profile of the child's communication skills in all environments as perceived by those who know him best, can begin to be formulated.

EDUCATION HISTORY

For the child at school it is most important for the therapist to seek information from the child's teacher about how he copes with the rather more demanding environment of the classroom. The way in which a child behaves in the classroom and how he relates to his peer group and adults outside the immediate family yields information about his understanding of social rules governing behaviour and social interaction. Similarly, the way a child approaches a new task or situation and his curiosity about the variety of materials available to him at school and his use of such materials will provide important information. There may be certain activities in which he will choose to participate, and indeed particular children with whom he will choose to play. There may be some things that he is particularly good at and some he is not. The child's ability to understand the rules of social interaction in a group and the language of the classroom is imperative if he is to cope with what he is expected to do. Only then can he make progress through the stages of the National Curriculum and develop rewarding social relationships with other children and adults.

The child's teacher will be able to tell the therapist about the child at school and describe his strengths and weaknesses across a range of learning situations and subjects. She will have invaluable information about the type of activities which appear to most interest the child and those which stimulate the child to use the language he has. The teacher will also have information about the child's individual learning patterns which will be essential to the intervention programme.

Methods of assessment

The speech and language therapist is trained in a variety of assessment methods and techniques and during the assessment period, both initially and during the course of therapy, will use a combination of such methods to ascertain the nature and extent of the child's difficulties and make a diagnosis. Account will be taken of the child's past experience as outlined in the case history. It is important to recognise that the information gained from assessment changes as the therapist gets to know the child and, of course, as the child becomes more familiar with the therapist and the clinical setting. The child presenting with a more complex speech and language difficulty would normally be assessed in a variety of settings including the clinic, classroom and often at home.

Many parents may be anxious about assessment and its implications for diagnosis and the resulting recommendations. Sometimes parents may feel that the result of the assessment is unrepresentative of the child's real abilities, and that if it had been presented in a different way, or done in a different place on a different day, that the result would also be different. Discussion about assessment between the therapist and parent is always necessary and some anxiety can be relieved by explaining exactly why the child failed a certain test item or responded inappropriately, and demonstrating other means to facilitate the child's understanding to help him succeed. Indeed, the child may well be having an 'off day' and it may be that it would be more appropriate to carry out the assessment at a different time. You should make sure that you tell the therapist if you think that this is the case when your child is assessed.

Generally assessment can be divided into informal and formal techniques for gathering the required information necessary to make a diagnosis. Both methods of assessment have inherent strengths and weaknesses, and the mode and variety of assessment tools used can be selected according to the individual child and his presenting difficulties.

Informal assessment

This type of assessment will include information gathering techniques both direct and indirect. Direct information gathering in the form of a detailed case history from parents has already been discussed. Therapists will also have documented their discussions with the child's teachers and have information related to his functioning within the classroom and his level of educational attainment with regard to the stages of the National Curriculum. Similarly, she may have sought information from other involved agencies such as a paediatrician, educational psychologist or audiologist.

Initially, the therapist is likely to engage the child in play and conversation with toys or materials appropriate to his age and preference, to begin indirect informal assessment. Parents will usually be actively encouraged to participate in the child's play to enable the therapist to observe the child interacting and using language with a familiar adult and thus begin to evaluate the child's present range of skills which are relevant to the development of speech and language. With younger children the therapist may well play on the floor with a variety of toys specifically chosen to elicit given responses. For example, she may choose a shape sorter to see if the child can manipulate and match the shapes appropriately. Commonly, she will use large dolls, teddies and toy-size furniture to see how the child relates to these objects and how sophisticated his play and language are when engaged in these activities.

During this 'play time' the therapist will be building rapport with the child, finding out what he is interested in and testing various skills through the choice of equipment and language used. For example, she may ask the child to 'give the teddy a drink' to help ascertain whether or not he can understand the specific vocabulary used, and the specific instruction given. Many children in this situation will spontaneously give a drink to a toy or adult, but may fail to respond to a specific verbal request such as the above through lack of verbal understanding. During such informal assessment sessions the therapist will be using the knowledge she has of normal child development and in particular the development of attention and listening skills, play skills, social interaction skills and the development of speech and language to 'test out' the child's abilities and identify areas of difficulty which need further assessment. She will also be identifying particular areas of strength or skill, which can be used during therapy. Assessment of this type is continuous and each time the child and therapist meet she will be re-evaluating the child's performance, comparing it to the initial findings and planning for the future sessions accordingly.

Formal assessment

Formal assessment involves the use of tests which follow a set procedure. The person administering the test must use particular wording for questions and often makes use of a given set of materials. The tester is looking for specific responses. Some parents are concerned that their child could have performed better if the question had been asked in a different way. However, rewording a question can mean that the test result is invalidated. The advantage of such formal procedures is that the results can be compared with other children of the same age. Similarly, the same child can be assessed on a number of occasions and the results compared over-time.

Many such tests are developed on a 'normal' population. This allows us to work out standard scores. These will show how near or far away from 'the norm', or what is expected and achieved by most children of that age, the child is. Such scoring systems have limitations, and it is not always helpful to compare children in this way, particularly children from bilingual homes for whom such tests are often inappropriate. The 'age equivalent score' which can also be obtained from this test, gives parents and therapists an idea of the 'language age' level the child has reached. For example, a child of five years six months who achieves a raw score of 51 (i.e. passed 51 items) on the verbal comprehension (or understanding) section of the Reynell Developmental Language Scales will, when calculations are made using a set of tables, achieve an equivalent age of four years. This means that although his chronological age is five years six months, the language concepts he is able to understand are more like those of a child of four.

A number of such tests are available. They are used in conjunction with other informal techniques and methods of assessment and help provide invaluable information necessary to reach a diagnosis and plan appropriate therapeutic intervention. Speech and language therapists are specially trained to administer and interpret a battery of tests which may not be available to other professionals for use, and to interpret and evaluate the results of such tests in consideration of the individual child, his individual circumstances and his responses on that particular day.

There is much discussion about 'one-off' testing of children. Necessarily, all assessments have strengths and weaknesses and the type of information gleaned from such a test would only be a part of the picture the therapist is trying to formulate of the child's skills. The vast majority of the tests available for use with younger children consist of toys and picture materials with which most children would be familiar, and often keen to play with. In the event that the child is uncooperative and not willing to participate in the test situation, the way the child manages this situation, whatever he chooses to do instead, is important. How he plays with materials offered and the language he is understanding and using to express his non-compliance will yield useful information for the therapist. Tests for older children, such as the Clinical Evaluation of Language Fundamentals – Revised (CELF–R), consist of a battery of pictures and verbal instructions, graded in complexity. This tests a range of linguistic structures (e.g. ability to understand plurals, concepts of time, identify words with similar meaning and his ability to formulate appropriate spoken responses to a variety of questions, pictures etc).

Among the tests most commonly used in the UK are the Reynell Developmental Language Scales, the Lowe and Costello Symbolic Play Test, the CELF–R, the Derbyshire Language Scheme, the Test of Reception of Grammar and the Renfrew Bus Story. Each of these tests looks at different aspects of the child's communicative competence and in the case of the Symbolic Play Test, the ability of the child to use miniature toys in a representational way, which is a necessary pre-cursor to language development and a useful indication of present levels of cognitive functioning.

The Reynell Developmental Language Scales, for example, is divided into two sections dealing with verbal comprehension and expression, respectively, and can be used with children between the ages of one and seven years. The comprehension section comprises ten sub-tests involving listening to a verbal instruction and carrying out a command using toys:

e.g. materials: pencil, knife, saucepan, bed, broom.

Instructions to child, where child is required to point:

'Which one can you sleep in?'

'Which one can you write with?' etc.

This section, which tests a child's understanding of a range of instructions, graded in complexity, does not require the child to make any verbal response. Gesture, pointing and 'eye' pointing are sufficient. There is a section designed to test 'expressive language' or spoken language skills. It looks at the child's abilities to name objects and respond to simple and complicated pictures. The tester is also expected to make an assessment of the child's use of grammar. The total number of correct responses for both sections is scored independently and translated to an age equivalent and then a standard score.

Other commonly used assessments include those associated with the Derbyshire Language Scheme. These are known as the Rapid Screening Test and the Detailed Test of Comprehension. Both use toys, everyday objects and picture materials. As in the case of the Reynell Developmental Language Scales, the child's verbal comprehension is tested by asking him to complete a task by following a verbal instruction from the tester, e.g. 'Put the teddy on the bed.' However, the instructions are more carefully graded in complexity ranging from simple requests such as 'show me the shoe', when presented with four clear pictures of everyday objects, to complex instructions such as 'put the pencil on the plate and close the purse' carried out with real objects. The number of items passed in this test and the ultimate scoring is described in terms of 'information carrying word levels' and then translated to an age-range equivalent. For example, a two-year-old would be expected to carry out commands containing two important ideas or words, i.e. a 'two information carrying word level', e.g. 'put the *shoes* on the *bed*', when there is a greater choice of things to do with them or other toys/objects which could be used if the specific words and request are not understood. A two-year-old with memory and attention difficulties may not respond at all, or simply point to the bed. The assessments associated with the Derbyshire Language Scheme are particularly useful in identifying specific areas of weakness or gaps in development which the child is experiencing, and thus form the basis for many language programmes and future therapeutic intervention or teaching.

Therapists often use tape recordings or transcripts of the child's utterances during free play to obtain a 'language sample'. A number of different analyses can be carried out on these samples – e.g. looking at the grammatical structures the child is using or analysing the child's development of speech sounds. Expressive language skills are more often observed and analysed by the therapist in a range of settings – clinic, classroom, home – where social interaction skills and the ability to use language meaningfully and with purpose, to be understood by others, are more the focus of assessment. The therapist may present the child with a range of materials and conversational situations either on his own, or with a small group of other children at school, to elicit certain responses and prompt particular forms of social interaction and relevant accompanying language.

For example, a child may at first appear at school to be a lively chatterbox and frequent contributor to classroom talk. Upon observation and analysis such a child may be understanding little of others' language and may be unaware of the rules of conversation governing social interaction, i.e. he may not listen to others, he may not be able to take turns, he may only be able to talk about his favourite topics and be unaware of, or unable to repair, a breakdown in conversation.

Some children have, for example, difficulties remembering words – a condition sometimes known as *specific word finding difficulties*. They have an inability to retrieve a specific word from the memory store when required, and may have stilted and empty conversation. Parents sometimes talk of their children 'going round the houses'. Therapists call this *circumlocuting*. For example in describing a picture:

milkman – the, er, that man with, the pint-man;

umbrella – put it in the sky and you know, for raining;

The child will find specific naming tasks very difficult and this type of naming activity will help the therapist identify such problems and plan to strengthen the child's retrieval skills and teach coping strategies through a variety of therapeutic techniques and teaching targets. When the therapist is satisfied that she has a general idea of the child's level of functioning with regard to speech and language development, she may wish to assess several areas in depth.

Other areas of development commonly assessed

There are six areas of the development of speech and language that therapists will wish to assess in particular, and any of those areas in which the child appears to be having particular difficulty will be assessed in depth.

Attention and listening

As with other developmental skills such as learning to sit independently, to wash, to hold a pencil in a mature tripod grip, attention and listening skills similarly follow a predictable developmental pattern. Many children with speech and language difficulties have accompanying difficulties in focusing and maintaining attention to a task or to language. They may also have problems with listening selectively to relevant auditory stimuli and in developing sophisticated listening skills which enable children to carry on working or playing while at the same time listening to verbal commentary or instructions.

Clinicians will ask parents and teachers which activities or situations best hold the child's attention. When she has observed the child she will be able to compare the development of his attention and listening skills to those of other children.

Children with attention and listening difficulties often experience great difficulty in learning. They often fail to complete tasks, e.g. a puzzle, a drawing and listening to a short story, and flit from activity to activity unless focused by an adult. This interferes with the opportunity for learning by repeated experience and practice. Similarly, such difficulties will limit the amount of verbal information the child can process and this may affect the number of opportunities he will have to learn the meaning of language.

Play

Children's play also follows a discernable developmental pattern. In babies, play is exploratory – mouthing, feeling and banging objects. Many of a baby's apparently random movements, say of the hands, result in a response. She may, for example, accidentally hit a mobile while waving her hands around. The reaction will probably precipitate a repetition of the movement. Adults will then say that she is playing with her mobile.

Similarly, children move through other developmental stages of play:

exploratory – picks up brush, fingers it, mouths it, pushes it.

relational – brushes own hair, brushes doll.

representational – uses props to stand for brush, scissors, rollers etc.

symbolic – pretend hairdresser scenes.

The therapist will observe the child in free play with family members or peers. She will also use specific play materials in the clinic to facilitate the child in demonstrating his play skills. Toy dolls, teddies, cups, plates, spoons and beds are used in many clinics and schools. These items are usually familiar to children and they generally enjoy playing with them. The way in which children play with such materials is of particular interest to the therapist because of the link already mentioned between symbolic play, cognitive development and the development of language. For example children of different ages use toys quite differently. A 12-month-old will mouth a brick or throw it while a four-year-old may put it together with other bricks, making a tower or turn it into something more exciting such as a car or a helicopter.

A formal play test, the Lowe and Costello Symbolic Play Test may also be used in assessment. This test consists of a number of miniature toys with which the child is encouraged to play. The therapist will observe the child's responses and the way in which he uses the toys, and score expected responses on a scoring sheet. A total will be obtained which converts to a standard score (see Glossary).

As the child gets older it becomes more difficult to test symbolic play. How much can we know about what a child is thinking when they are using a toy, for example? But also, of course, as children move into school their play becomes more a matter of how they interact with their peers rather than what they do with specific toys. Speech and language therapists are very interested in how children play with others in their family and their class and will often spend periods of time observing activities that the child is engaged in. It is interesting that many children with delayed speech or language choose to play with children younger than their age. This is probably because the interactions are less complicated and less verbally demanding and this makes it easier for them to cope socially.

Verbal comprehension

The development of verbal comprehension follows a prescribed path and can be measured and compared to norms for a given age group or developmental stage. Difficulties with verbal comprehension are extremely common in children referred for speech and language therapy. The degree of difficulty varies in severity and its impact upon the child's ability to use expressive language and learn from the classroom curriculum can be profound. Similarly, such difficulties can lead to frustration and 'behaviour problems', and some children with significant difficulties in understanding language may be described as 'naughty', 'difficult to manage' or 'solitary'. It is important to recognise that parents sometimes do not realise that their child has difficulty understanding. They may simply have got used to speaking to him at a simpler level than would be expected for his age. Of course, the same can be true of teachers. Often, the focus of school activities is what the child actually says, what is known as his *verbal output* or *verbal expression*, and it is his difficulty in using expressive language and the way he speaks that has prompted concern and referral to the speech and language therapist.

Parents', teachers' and therapists' notion of what we mean by verbal understanding, varies. By *verbal understanding* the speech and language therapist means the ability to know what a spoken word means, to remember that word, to differentiate that word from similar words (either in meaning: coat, shoe; or sound: cap, cat), and to understand the meaning of the word in isolation, where there are no contextual, gestural or other non-verbal clues. For example, a teacher may feel that the child understands classroom instructions because he follows the class routine, lining up at appropriate times, knowing where things go at tidying-up time, taking the register to the office. On assessment, where the routine is changed and there are no clues given by the teacher/parent or therapist, it may be evident that the child does not, in fact, understand such verbal commands. The child who cannot follow a 'test command' in the clinic of 'give me the pencil and the book' where there are no classroom distractions, would not be able to understand a more complex, but common classroom command of 'go and get the tin of pencils from Laurie's table then get your number book and sit with Ms Silver', but may comply with such a request at school simply because it is routine, in context and accompanied by gesture.

Therapists will use a variety of techniques to assess the level of the child's understanding of language. They will often ask parents and teachers about situations in which the child seems to cope and conversely situations in which the child relies on other information – gesture, context and routine – to work out what is going on. For example some children will always wait until last when the class has been given an instruction so that they can copy other children and not have to rely on understanding a verbal instruction.

Verbal expression

A child's 'output' or expressive language, also follows a predictable developmental pattern. The therapist will apply her skills and knowledge to ascertain the type and range of language used by the child in terms of syntax, vocabulary, semantics and use of language. Through assessment and observation she will build a profile of each of the above and look at how they interact.

This information will establish a 'base-line' of the child's expressive language skills and enable the therapist to plan the intervention programme accordingly. She will have been able to identify strengths and weaknesses in the child's verbal output. Some of the methods used for ascertaining this information have already been described. For example, many language-impaired children have difficulty learning to use words and many have a poorly developed vocabulary. However, the grammatical rules we apply in English or indeed in other languages, to place classes or types of words in particular places within a sentence, may be developing normally.

Thus a child may say in response to a picture of a child drawing: 'she's doing a thing', where the information supplied would be clearly inadequate to convey an idea or message without the usual clue of the picture. This is only one example of a type of language difficulty that the therapist will be looking for, or ruling out as part of the problem. As the child gets older he often continues to have difficulty forming sentences and continues to simplify what he says. In many cases this simply makes him sound like a younger child. However, there are cases where what the child says makes it very difficult to follow exactly what he means. For example if he continually uses pronouns (eg: *he, she, it, they*) rather than using the relevant nouns it can be very difficult to ascertain who he is talking about or to what he is referring. Equally if he misses out prepositions such as *off, out, on* etc., his use of a given verb can be very imprecise. Thus he might say 'He jumped the bus' do we know whether he means he jumped '*off*' or '*on to*' or even '*under*' the bus? Of course, with younger children we do not expect such precision and make all sorts of judgements from the context. But the child of seven or eight would not be expected to make such mistakes and it can lead to all sorts of misunderstandings. A parent or teacher may then ask the child to clarify what they have said and the child has to *repair* the conversation, in other words to make his intended meaning clear. For many language-impaired children such repairs are difficult because they in themselves may require a high level of fluency.

Speech

The speech and language therapist draws the distinction between speech – phonology and articulation – and language – grammar, vocabulary, semantics and pragmatics – or use of language. Many children referred to speech and language therapists have difficulties with speech and, as with language difficulties, the range and severity vary enormously. Assessments for speech delay or disorder generally consist of an oral examination and an analysis of a spontaneous speech sample taken from a tape recording of spontaneous or elicited speech. Elicited speech samples will target particular sounds and combinations of sounds, – from single vowel and consonant sounds, to single words, polysyllabic words, phrases and sentences. There are several assessments available for use including the Edinburgh Articulation Test, the Nuffield Dyspraxia Assessment, Metaphon, the South Tyneside Assessment of Phonological Processes, and Phonological Assessment of Child Speech (PACS). All such assessments use picture materials to elicit a specific response and yield results both in forms of 'age levels' and identification of the inventory of single sounds a child can produce and their proximity to the adult model and phonological processes the child is using.

The speech and language therapist will look carefully at the child's ability to use and coordinate the muscles required for speech. The oral examination will consist of testing a number of oral movements, e.g. range and accuracy and palate, tongue, lip movements, breathing and the ability to carry out a purposeful act, for example, protrusion of the tongue, on command.

The speech sample elicited spontaneously and through testing will be transcribed phonetically and then analysed phonologically to look at the range of sounds used, the systems the child is using and the contrasts he can make between sounds (e.g. /k/ and /t/ or /g/ and /d/). Through assessment the therapist will be able to identify any one or more of a number of processes the child is using, some of which may be simply immature or delayed speech patterns, and others of which may be disordered, and not following a normal developmental pattern.

Social interaction and use of language

The way in which children learn the rules of social interaction and how to use language has already been referred to in Chapter 2. It is indeed remarkable that the majority of children acquire such sophisticated methods of communicating and can use many social and linguistic nuances so early and in such a short space of time.

However, in some children these skills do not develop adequately as they may have particular difficulties which have a considerable impact upon the development of social relationships – both within the family and in the wider community. In school it will impact upon their ability to access the National Curriculum and make progress through its prescribed stages. More important, children with difficulties in use of language may fail to make rewarding, social relationships with their peers and may not readily be able to participate in group discussions and group or cooperative learning.

Again, the speech and language therapist will use her knowledge of the development of interaction, and the way in which people speak to one another, together with a variety of checklists and assessment materials to describe the quality and range of language functions the child uses.

Such skills may vary widely with the situation in which the assessment takes place and in the majority of cases the therapist will need to see the child in a range of natural settings, such as at home and school, as well as the clinic. There are few formal assessments to help us look at these skills, probably because it is so difficult to specifically elicit some of these behaviours. The one scale that is commonly used in the UK is the Pragmatics Profile. This is administered in the form of an interview and focuses on a number of areas of communication. The therapist would commonly address the questions to the person who knows the child best – usually the parent or the teacher.

Summary

When you first go to a speech and language therapy appointment it can be quite a daunting experience. This chapter has gone some way towards explaining the type of questions you will be asked and the kind of assessments that will be carried out. However, as we noted in Chapter 2, many of these children will also need to be seen by other professionals and it is to them that we turn now.

CHAPTER 4

What Else Can He Do?
The View of Other Professionals

Many children who experience difficulties learning speech and language may be immature in other areas. As a result it is important that these other areas are assessed thoroughly. The pattern of strengths and weaknesses is a puzzle which parents and professionals have to solve together. In this chapter we turn to the four professionals who are most likely to be involved with your child: the paediatrician, the psychologist, the physiotherapist and the occupational therapist.

The paediatrician
Sundara Lingam, paediatrician

Children are seen by health visitors, clinic doctors or general practitioners at specified times for health and development tracking. This is usually referred to as *child health surveillance*. As part of this surveillance procedure the health visitor is also involved in health promotion which includes encouraging the prevention of accidents and illness. They also inform parents about nutrition and the need for immunisation. Most health visitors and doctors involved in child health surveillance use a parental questionnaire to elicit information to supplement their observations. Sometimes parents are asked to fill in such questionnaires before they come to the appointment. A child's development is always then related to what we know about normal development.

The role of the paediatrician

For convenience, development is assessed in a number of areas:

1. Gross motor

2. Fine motor

3. Vision

4. Hearing

5. Speech and language

6. Social development

7. Play.

About 20 per cent of children give cause for concern because of their development and would need a more detailed examination by a paediatrician (a specialist in children's health and development). This is usually carried out at a child development centre (CDC). Here the child will also typically be seen by a range of other professionals including the speech and language therapist, the physiotherapist and the occupational therapist. The members of the CDC team are usually more experienced and specialised in child development. Liaison with families is also carried out by specialist health visitors and social workers. Not all child development teams include all the different professionals nor is it necessary for every child referred to the CDC to be seen by them all.

The paediatrician in the CDC would take a detailed family history covering areas such as the pregnancy, the labour, the delivery and feeding in early life. There are various patterns of development which the paediatrician will be looking for.

NORMAL VARIATION IN DEVELOPMENT

Some children progress more slowly than others in one area of their development. For example they may be late in walking but normal in other areas. This type of behaviour may run in the family. Such children will normally be kept under observation by the paediatrician in the child health clinic.

EARLY ONSET DEVELOPMENTAL DELAY

Such children would have progressed slowly in all parameters of development from very early on in life. All developmental milestones will be affected.

LATE ONSET DEVELOPMENTAL DELAY

This is usually identified by parents but confirmed by the paediatrician. It is characterised by normal early milestones, after which development starts to slow down. This may be caused by illness but, as often as not, the cause is unknown.

REGRESSION

In such cases the child usually would have developed normally and the health record would clearly show that there were no concerns. However, at some stage, the child stops progressing and as he grows older even begins to lose skills. This is a worrying problem not only for the family but for the paediatrican and all the other team members. Regression has several possible causes.

Examination and investigation

Every child attending the CDC will have a *neuro developmental examination* in addition to a full physical examination. The paediatrician will arrange for the child's height and weight to be measured. Particular attention will be paid to the child's head size. If a child has a very large or a very small head the paediatrician might also measure the head size of the parents or the other children in the family. Similarly if a child looks 'different' for any reason, the paediatrician will record all the abnormalities. Features of this type are known as 'dysmorphic' ('dys' meaning different, 'morphic' refers to appearance – i.e. of unusual appearance). For example, the doctor will look at hair pattern, eyes, neck, ears, palate and so on. They also inspect the child's hands and feet looking for any difference in the size or for any abnormal skin creases.

Chromosomal defects are the usual cause of dysmorphism, but a small number of children might have other explanations; such as infection of the baby in the womb or the effects of anticonvulsant drugs or other medication taken by the mother during pregnancy. Similarly drinking alcohol to excess during pregnancy can lead to the birth of a dysmorphic baby which is developmentally delayed (foetal alcohol syndrome). Paediatricians will also look carefully at the child's skin for white or dark patches which may also be associated with developmental difficulties. The paediatrician will also, of course, arrange for a hearing test to be carried out, if this has not already been done.

It is the duty of paediatricians to organise and explain the tests which they are arranging. The paediatrician will also discuss the results with the parents as soon as they come back from the laboratory. If the results are *positive* this means that the test has identified a problem. Sometimes test results such as the chromosome test can take a long time to come through. The following investigations may be arranged.

BLOOD CHROMOSOME TEST

Every human has 46 chromosomes (23 pairs). The baby gets 23 from the father and 23 from the mother. Sometimes, following the fertilisation of the egg, the foetus may develop a small but significant chromosome defect. Breakage (deletion), additions or omissions are the most common problems. *Down's Syndrome* babies have an additional chromosome (47). Some boys and girls who show delays in all areas of their development may have a breakage in the X (sex) chromosome. This is called the *Fragile X Syndrome*. Such children may have a range of learning difficulties and associated speech and language problems and are likely to need special help.

BLOOD TESTS

These are used to check a number of functions. For example, they can help ascertain whether there is a problem with the thyroid gland or muscle enzymes called Creative Phosphokinase (CPK). Children with thyroid deficiency often show developmental delays. Similarly, boys who have muscular dystrophy may present with developmental delay and it is therefore important that this is checked for by doing muscle enzyme tests. Liver function tests and immunoglobulin tests may also be carried out.

URINE AMINOACIDS, ORGANIC ACIDS, AND PH TESTING

These are carried out to ensure that the child's problems are not due to some abnormal chemical in the child which is the cause of the child's developmental delay.

LUMBAR PUNCTURE

Some children need a lumbar puncture to study the fluid which surrounds the brain (the cerebro-spinal fluid or CSF). This might show that the child has an encephalitis. Children who contract the rubella virus in the womb typically have abnormal CSF.

X-RAYS

These are carried out to examine the child's bone structure. They are used to detect damage to the bones and joints but may also help in identifying children who have advanced bone age, another phenomenon which may point to a specific diagnosis.

BRAIN SCANS

Electrophysiological tests such as electroencephalopathy (EEG) are used to monitor activity in the brain. They are still used relatively rarely but may help in identifying brain malformation or brain damage in cases where a child has epilepsy. Recently, considerable strides have been made in what are known as brain imaging techniques. Of these, one in particular, known as Magnetic Resonance Imaging (MRI), looks as if it may help us understand more about the structure of the brain and which areas are used for which purposes. It is unclear as yet to what extent it will help us treat individual children.

Liaison

This is a major task for the paediatrician involved in child development. The paediatrician must explain the diagnosis and its implications to parents/carers – a task which is often very hard. The child development team as a whole must also be prepared to share their thoughts and concerns with parents. All the findings are written down clearly after discussion with the rest of the CDC team. It is customary for parents to receive a copy of the report. Parents can always ask for a copy of the report if this is not the usual practice in the CDC that they attend. The team will also give information about voluntary organisations which can offer support. The paediatrician will encourage the parents to attend follow-up appointments.

The paediatrician has responsibility for the child's health but if the problem concerns housing or education there is often relatively little that the paediatrician can do. Housing issues are dealt with by the Housing and Social Services and decisions on educational matters are ultimately made by the education authority. The paediatrician would, however, be able to write to the education or Housing and Social Services to express concern and help support parental concerns where appropriate. He will help with applications for rehousing on medical grounds, or help from social services on the grounds of the child's special needs.

Paediatricians also have a duty under the 1981 Education Act to notify the education authority of any child (at any age) who is in need of special provision in education. For example if a child of three years shows an overall developmental delay, it is best to send notification of this child to the education department. This is known as a Section 176 notification. The aim is to let the education department, who, after all, have responsibility for the education of the child, know that the child might need help now or later on. The earlier the education department knows about the child the earlier the most appropriate educational provision can be offered.

Under the Children Act, social services must keep a register of all clients with a disability. It is the duty of the CDC team and the paediatrician or the specialist social worker to explain the need for this and, with parental consent, notify the social services about the child. If the parents agree for their child to be on the disability register it becomes easier for appropriate services to be planned and offered.

Finally, paediatricians like other professionals are there to do all they can to help the child and family. Parents and children have a right to know what is needed and parents are encouraged to ask questions, and yet more questions, about their child. If they are unhappy with the answers that they receive they must ask the paediatrician to refer their child for a second opinion from another doctor or CDC team.

The psychologist
Roger Penniceard, educational psychologist

Children with speech and language problems have usually been assessed and often treated by a speech and language therapist for a period before the start of a statementing procedure. As a result of this intervention a considerable amount is often already known about the child's abilities and problems. However, it is a statutory part of the statementing procedure that the child is seen by an educational psychologist who, unlike the speech and language therapist, is an employee of the education authority.

The role of the psychologist

There is often confusion between psychologists and psychiatrists. A psychiatrist is a medical doctor who has specialised in treating emotional and behavioural problems. A psychologist is not medically trained, but in doing a degree in psychology she has studied how man (and animals) develop, learn, communicate, think; how we observe and understand the world, what motivates us and how we interact socially. Behavioural and emotional problems form a part of that study and this is the area in which the role of the psychologist overlaps with that of the psychiatrist. Those psychologists who wish to work primarily with this aspect would do further training and become clinical psychologists. Those graduates who are interested in children and how they learn and develop would follow a different training route and become educational psychologists. To do this they will have a teaching qualification and will have taught for at least two years before doing a training course in educational psychology.

In assessing a child the educational psychologist is trying to get a picture of the child's development and the factors which have influenced it, such as the environment, illness or accident and the family. The Code of Practice on the Identification and Assessment of Special Educational Needs says that the psychologist should look at the 'child's cognitive functioning; communication skills; perceptual and motor skills; adaptive and personal and social skills; the child's attitudes and approaches to learning; his or her educational attainments; and the child's self-image, interests and behaviour'. The aim of this process is to determine what is required to optimise the child's educational progress. What the psychologist will have to do in a particular situation will vary depending on the age of the child and what information is already available. Thus, not all of the steps discussed will be necessary on every occasion.

The psychologist will want to look at the child's skills in a variety of areas to determine how well he or she is doing relative to what would be expected at the child's age. In order to do this the psychologist may use what are called standardised tests (see Chapter 3 for further discussion).

A description of how these tests are developed and what they are attempting to do may provide us with an insight into the type of information they give. Initially a number of different tasks are selected which involve a wide range of skills. These are then given to a large number of children. The children are chosen so that they are representative of the population in terms of social class, ethnic background etc. When a child is tested it is being compared with this group of children. In order to ensure that each child who does the test has an equal chance of success, the items are presented in a carefully specified way. It is this aspect which sometimes causes frustration when parents watch children doing this type of test, because they feel that if the task was presented in a slightly different way the child would be able to succeed. This is especially the case when children with language problems are being asked questions. It is very difficult for parents to refrain from rephrasing the question in a way which they know will be more understandable to the child, but it is important that the psychologist does the task in the recommended way so that the child can be compared validly to the standardisation sample (the large number of other children to whom the test was initially given). Having done the test in the standard way, sometimes a psychologist may modify the presentation to explore why the child is having difficulty.

There are arguments both for and against parents being present during this type of formal assessment. Ultimately it is important that the child is able to work as well as possible. A very young child may feel more confident with a parent, but an older child may be inhibited. It is more usual for the psychologist to see the child on its own, but this is something that can be discussed.

Parents are often worried, especially with younger children, that the child will not cooperate or will have an 'off day'. The psychologist will be prepared for this eventuality and will have a number of ways of dealing with the situation and getting the necessary information. For example, a considerable amount of information can be obtained from the parent using carefully structured questionnaires. An experienced psychologist is not dependent on formal tests. Many of the test items are similar to toys. By watching what the child does with toys and other objects around the house or classroom, a lot of valuable information can be gained. The psychologist may spend time playing on the floor with the child. Even when formal tests are attempted and the child does not cooperate, the child may often subsequently play with the materials while the psychologist is talking to the parent and in doing so will provide the required information. In situations where the psychologist knows beforehand that the child finds new situations and strangers difficult, various strategies may be used. For example, the psychologist may arrange to do the assessment in the child's normal speech therapy session with the therapist.

The psychologist is interested in observing the child solving puzzles, remembering, reasoning, drawing, copying, answering questions etc. The type of test which provides a structured way of doing such a wide-ranging observation is an intelligence test. It must be stressed that the psychologist is interested in observing the child working on a wide range of tasks, not in merely deriving a measure of the child's intelligence. However, at the end of the assessment the psychologist may make a general comment about the child's ability.

In addition to important observations as to how the child related and dealt with the situation and the tasks, the psychologist will have a number of scores which reflect how well the child did on each of the tests. Like IQ figures, these scores can easily be misinterpreted, thus psychologists are often reluctant to put the figures into reports. The scores on the verbal parts of the intelligence test, if they were done, may be very poor, but this of course does not mean that the child is unintelligent. How the child dealt with these tests and the scores obtained may reflect something of the extent of the child's speech and language problem and will have given the psychologist an opportunity to see how well the child understands, and to hear the child using language. This first-hand information, combined with the more specialised assessment of the speech and language therapist, will be used by the psychologist in other parts of the assessment and to formulate the child's needs.

Intelligence tests usually have a number of sub-tests which do not directly involve language. These are called *non-verbal* or *performance* tests. Such things as drawing, jigsaw puzzles, sorting, picture matching, picture sequencing and copying patterns are examples of non-verbal tests. Unfortunately the standard procedure for using many of these tests requires the use of verbal instructions. In many cases the child can understand enough of what is being said, in the context of a demonstration, to be able to do the task. Nevertheless, the psychologist has to judge whether the child's performance on any test item has been compromised by not understanding the instructions or whether the task has been made easier because it was necessary to give a more explicit visual demonstration of what was required. In situations where the child's language problems are severe, the psychologist may use a specialist test which has been designed to be presented completely non-verbally. Usually such tests have been designed for use with the deaf.

Mention has been made earlier that psychologists often do not quote test results because they are so easily misinterpreted, but when they are given they can be presented in a variety of ways. Before considering these, it should be stressed that when the child attempts a variety of different tasks some variation in the child's scores is expected, but these variations do not indicate strengths and weaknesses unless these differences are quite large. Where significant differences exist, the psychologist will have commented about the fact in the report, because this information may be used to advise teachers as to the best way to work with the child.

With young children, the results are often given in terms of ages. Consider, for example, remembering strings of digits. An adult would be expected to remember an eight or nine figure telephone number without difficulty; a child of five would be able to manage four digits, but a three-year-old would only be able to remember two reliably. A five-year-old who could only remember two digits would be said to be functioning at a three-year-old level. This is not an uncommon finding with children with language problems. However, age scores can be misleading. It might be expected that a result of say three years six months on a drawing test would be followed by three years seven months if the child got the next item correct, and so on, but the gradation is often very uneven. The next test item on many drawing tests is at a four year six month level. The child therefore does not have the opportunity of getting any result between three years six months and four years six months. The parent, seeing a set of age scores around four years three months and a drawing test score of three years six months might feel there was a problem with the child's drawing skills, when in fact the result is an artifact of the test.

Another way of presenting the results is as percentiles or centiles. A child with a score at the sixtieth centile would have done better than 59 per cent of children. The most common way of recording scores for older children is in terms of scaled scores. These are based on a statistical process. The average score is 10, and 50 per cent of children will get scaled scores of 8 to 12. Scaled scores of 16 and above or 4 and below are relatively rare and represent the top and bottom two per cent of the ability range.

Liaison

Having completed the assessment, the psychologist will discuss the results and the child's needs with the parent, but will not recommend a particular school or unit. This decision will be taken by the LEA in consultation with the parents, after a draft statement has been produced. The psychologist will subsequently write a report which will be seen by the parents along with other professional reports when they receive the draft statement. In some cases the report may be made available to parents before the draft statement is completed.

The educational psychologist has a key role in coordinating the professional information for the LEA, in drafting the child's needs and formulating ways in which the child can be helped to have full access to the National Curriculum. He or she also provides a link between the educational administration, the parent and the school, and may have a key role in reviewing the child's progress following completion of the assessment. Together, the parent and the psychologist can ensure that the child has the best opportunity to overcome any educational difficulties and is able to make full use of his or her abilities.

The physiotherapist
Sally Holt, physiotherapist

There are some children with speech and language disorders who also experience difficulties with their gross and fine motor abilities and they may be referred to a physiotherapist. In some cases the child may have been under the local child development centre from an early age and may well have had a routine physiotherapy assessment. However, there are many children whose difficulties do not become apparent until they have started school and the teacher and/or parent observe that the child is not as able as his peers. In these cases the school can refer the child directly for a physiotherapy assessment or the parent might mention the problems to the school doctor who will then make a referral. Ideally, the speech and language therapist involved with the child would be working as a part of a therapy team where cross referrals take place as a matter of course.

Often parents are aware that their child is not functioning physically quite as well as his siblings or his friends of a similar age, but the difficulties are often so subtle that it is hard to identify just what they are. Other parents, when asked if they have any concerns about their child's physical development will answer no, but as the assessment progresses they become aware of how much they have compensated for his difficulties without realising that they were doing so. This is perfectly normal and it often takes a person outside the family to suggest that perhaps the child is not functioning quite as well as he might.

The role of the physiotherapist

A physiotherapist assesses the physical ability of the child, observes what he can do and more importantly how he performs the movement. From the information gathered the physical problems can be identified and an appropriate plan of action is drawn up. In some cases this will involve the child having on-going treatment, but often the family is given an exercise programme to carry out on a regular basis, perhaps daily, and the child is reviewed in a few weeks time. Similarly, the physiotherapist will liaise with the child's special needs assistant or care assistant should they have this sort of help allocated at school.

The assessment

The majority of children whom the physiotherapist assesses have some basic skills such as being able to get down and up from the floor, walk and run, but their competence may be poor. This will affect their quality of movement and balance. Often they are described as having poor coordination and they may also have low muscle tone and weak joints. This means that their postural stability will be poor and this, in turn, will affect both *gross motor* and *fine motor* abilities. Muscle tone refers to the degree of tension in the muscle and its state of readiness to contract. In any assessment the following areas are covered and the physiotherapist then matches the answers to what she knows about normal development.

GROSS MOTOR

The following series of questions is geared towards trying to build up a picture of the child's gross motor skills.

- How far can the child walk?

- How does he manage on a shopping expedition or a day's outing?

- Does he tire easily – more than siblings at a similar age?

- Does he stumble or fall often?

- How does he manage in the play ground at school? Does he join in physical games with his peers?

- Does he enjoy playing with a ball, e.g. kicking a football?

- Does he manage in PE lessons? If not, what does he find difficult?

- Does he enjoy climbing on playground apparatus or is he very fearful?

- Does he ride a bike? Can he use pedals on a two wheeler? How long did it take him to learn these skills?

- What does he enjoy doing most?

- Can he manage stairs independently? Does he come down one at a time using alternate feet?

- Does he run, jump, skip and hop?

- How quickly can the child get up from the floor from lying on his back (two seconds is normal)?

FINE MOTOR

- Does he prefer to use one hand?

- Does he find writing difficult? Does he press too hard? Does he tire easily?

- How does he hold a pencil? Is it a mature grip or is it awkward?

- Can he use scissors?

- How well does he eat – e.g. using a fork and spoon or knife and fork? Can he cut food? Does he use his fingers given half a chance?

- Can he dress himself – do buttons, zips and laces?

- What does he play with? Can he manage both large and small Lego?

The physiotherapist would need to observe the child's concentration and whether he needs help to stay on task. Similarly, we need to know whether he has difficulty remaining seated in a chair. If there are obvious fine motor difficulties children may be referred to an occupational therapist.

In order for coordinated purposeful movement to take place the pelvic stability needs to be good. The centre of gravity of the human body is contained in this area and whatever position the body adopts it is essential for the centre of gravity to be fixed, so that the body weight can be adjusted correctly around it and the person remain balanced. This normally occurs automatically as we move from one position to another, and can be finely tuned as in the case of a dancer or an athlete.

However, some children lack the necessary stability of the pelvis and shoulder girdle and also often have low muscle tone. They tend to bear weight more on one side than the other and this can usually be observed when the child is lying down. Often one hip will be withdrawn to give the appearance of one leg being shorter than the other. Children do this in an effort to stabilise themselves. It means that they are reluctant to transfer weight freely and revolve the body around the centre of gravity when moving or trying complicated manoeuvres. In the end, they in fact de-stabilise themselves. This is a very subtle difficulty but can have a marked effect on the child's gross and fine motor skills. It also means that

the body is not working efficiently and that more effort ⸱
in balance and feel secure. As a result the child will fau.
the hands effectively it is necessary to have good shoulder g.
stability. If this is poorly developed the child may spend an
amount of energy stabilising himself some other way – for ex.
pressing his hand down when writing, jamming his elbows tightly agan.
the body etc. These tasks then become tiring in themselves and can mean
that the child is reluctant to continue and, in some cases, even try at all.

During the assessment the child's physical ability would be observed
in a range of positions. The physiotherapist will look to see whether the
child can get in and out of the position, whether he can maintain it and
then stay in balance while moving within the position. At the same time
strength and endurance of limbs and trunk would be evaluated and how
well the child bears his own weight will be closely observed. Assessment
of fine motor skills will often be carried out while the child is seated.

How can physiotherapy help?

Physiotherapy can be effective in improving gross and fine motor skills,
if a child carries out the appropriate exercise programme which may be
for no more than ten minutes a day. Usually the child will be supervised
by a parent or a special needs assistant with regular monitoring from the
physiotherapist. The physiotherapist will always tailor this programme to
each child's needs.

The occupational therapist
Liz Mathew and Ana Santo, occupational therapists

> Sam is a seven-year-old boy who has just spent another restless,
> sleepless night. His mum comes in to get his clothes ready and she
> leaves him to dress. She comes back shortly and, as usual, has to
> help him put his clothes on in the right way, and she always has to
> do up his buttons. As he has not learned to tie shoelaces, mum has
> resorted to using trainers with velcro tabs.
>
> At breakfast, Sam knocks his glass of milk over, has food all over
> his face and around his plate. In the bathroom, mum has to help
> him wipe up his face and he turns his face away from the flannel.
> As he prepares to leave, Sam and mum frantically look for his school

bag and its contents. Mum knows that Sam is a smart child, but is puzzled by all the difficulties he has at home doing simple things.

Sam has a hard time sitting and attending to the teacher at school. He doesn't like standing in lines, and prefers to be at the very back of one. Although he tries very hard, he needs help to finish an activity. His teacher has often noticed that he holds pencils and paint brushes as if they were strange objects. In the playground, Sam is usually by himself watching the other children. He sometimes joins in with running around, but avoids the swings, see-saws, and slides. His teacher is very concerned about Sam as he is a bright, cheerful child, who tries very hard.

Mum notices that he rarely plays with the toys in his room on return from school, preferring instead to watch television or play with his cars. At bedtime, Sam undresses and has a bath. He does not like showers as the spray tickles and feels strange. He climbs into bed, forgetting already that he has left his school bag in the front room.

Sam is typical of the kind of child referred to paediatric occupational therapy (OT). The types of problems that Sam exhibits are also sometimes found in children with speech and language difficulties. Children such as Sam are commonly referred to as being *clumsy* or awkward and from an early age parents are usually the first to notice that there is something different about their child's play or general abilities.

The role of the occupational therapist

OTs become involved with these children because of the difficulties they experience with practical everyday activities; that is, in dressing, eating, bathing, writing, drawing, using pencils/scissors in the classroom, playing with other children, exploring toys and using playground equipment. The OT's role is to investigate the underlying causes of the problems and provide intervention to facilitate maximum independence in all these situations.

The brain processes sensory information received from the skin (tactile), muscles and joints (proprioception), and balance receptors (vestibular) in the ear. When a child is playing in the playground he is using a lot of sensory information to guide his motor activities which helps him learn about the environment. As he plays on the swings, he gains information about where he is in space (up and off the ground), what his body is doing (sitting, pumping with his legs, holding the rope), and whether he is falling off or not (balance and movement). By playing on the swing the child has gained body awareness, learned about the movement he can make and where he is in space.

The assessment

The OT will analyse an activity to determine which aspects affect a child's abilities. It is generally considered that good sensory, motor, perceptual functions are the building blocks for the acquisition of complex skills; the child must be able to sit without falling over, rest his forearm on the table, hold the pencil correctly, and guide the pencil to draw or write. All such skills rely on sensory, motor and perceptual mechanisms working well together. The purpose of the OT assessment is to gain an understanding of sensory, motor and perceptual functioning and how they affect practical everyday tasks both at home and in nursery or school. Information is gathered by interviewing the parents about their child's development and performance at home, observing the child in play, when involved in specific activities, and through the use of standardised tests.

DEVELOPMENTAL PROFILE

The OT will ask questions about early developmental history:

- ° what was your child like as a baby and what is he like now? – content or irritable?

- ° what are his sleep patterns like?

- ° when compared to other children, was he more difficult to handle or fussy?

- ° when did he sit, roll, crawl and walk?

The above questions pertain to early sensory behaviours and are essential to building a profile of his abilities and difficulties. Research indicates that children with motor coordination problems are often irritable or passive babies. Many children with language impairment reach their motor milestones at the appropriate time, although parents often say later that they felt something was wrong at the time.

PLAY HISTORY

- ○ does he explore and manipulate toys?
- ○ does he enjoy imaginative or creative play?
- ○ does he enjoy or avoid messy play?
- ○ does he play with children older or younger than him?
- ○ does he share or take turns?

The OT is interested in finding out how he plays with toys in general and which toys he particularly enjoys. The child who does not manipulate Lego blocks will often play with cars, an activity which does not require so much dexterity. It is also important to know if he plays with other children. Some children who do not feel confident with play or motor skills, will often prefer to play with younger children, because they can meet the expectations of the younger age group.

SELF-CARE HISTORY

Self-care refers to those activities the child has to learn in order to take care of himself.

Eating/meal times

- ○ how does the child eat?
- ○ what cutlery does he use: spoon, fork, knife?
- ○ is he messy?

A lot of information will be asked relating to eating and in particular his ability to feed himself. The OT is interested in not only how he uses his hands, which will indicate the maturity of his motor skills, but also how he chews, swallows etc. The types of food he likes and dislikes will provide some insight into the level of maturity, and how his sensory system is working – especially touch. For example, some children do not like certain food textures, while others are not aware of the food being on their face. The OT will also observe how the child grips cutlery and uses his hands together.

Dressing

- ○ how does he put on and take off clothes?
- ○ how does he do up and undo buttons and zippers?

- ° how does he tie shoelaces?
- ° does he put on and take off clothes in the right order?
- ° does he tolerate the labels on the back of his shirt?
- ° does he prefer certain clothes and avoid others?

When asking your child to remove and put on his shirt, the OT is looking to see whether he puts on clothing in the correct sequence, and if he uses the small muscles in his hand to do up buttons, laces etc. Observation of dressing also gives us information about how he uses his body, arms, legs and balance to dress himself. Some children are fussy about the textures of the clothes they wear, or perhaps they find labels irritating. These observations would provide information on how he processes tactile information.

Bathing

- ° can he bath by himself?
- ° can he dry himself?
- ° does he like to take showers or baths?
- ° how does he dry himself?

To bath, a child must have good body awareness, organisation and coordination. Some children who are sensitive to touch, dislike the spray of showers and prefer baths. To dry himself, a child must be able to coordinate his movements to manoeuvre the towel and complete the task in an organised manner.

Personal care

The OT may ask you questions about your child's reaction to having his hair or nails cut. Research suggests that children who have difficulties processing tactile information are not very tolerant of these activities and will try to avoid them.

NURSERY/SCHOOL WORK

- ° how does he hold pencils, crayons, scissors?
- ° how is his handwriting: large, faint, reversed letters, poor spacing, messy?

- ○ can he finish an activity without reminders?

- ○ does he need help to organise his work and materials?

- ○ how does he sit at the table?

- ○ does he like messy play with sand, finger paint or glue?

Children like Sam need help to start and complete an activity. Through questions about motor skills, the OT is also trying to find out whether he has any difficulty in holding and/or using tools in a coordinated manner.

PLAYGROUND

- ○ does he ride a bike?

- ○ how does he stand on one leg, hop, skip, run?

- ○ does he enjoy or avoid certain playground equipment?

- ○ can he catch and/or throw a ball?

Not only do these questions relate to body awareness and coordination, but also to his emotional reactions (e.g., fear) to activities which require balance. Again, research suggests that these children who are sensitive to movement, avoid such activities and cannot make use of opportunities to develop these skills. This can become a vicious circle as a child does not learn to use the equipment and, as a result, does not develop other related skills.

DEVELOPMENTAL OBSERVATIONS

Developmental observations are made watching the child perform certain tasks during play, structured activities or standardised tests. Familiar toys (beads, pegs, crayons, scissors, ball, puzzles, paper, buttons etc.) are used to help the child feel more at home.

Standardised tests present another important opportunity for the OT to observe the child. The score is important for the team to gain an idea of the level of ability but, from an OT perspective, the quality of performance is also important. Observations made during the test may support what was seen during other activities and what the parents have reported. Test scores also provide a measure of his ability which can be used comparatively, especially following treatment.

Sensory: the OT looks for reactions to sensation which are inherent to the task. She may present specific tasks or tests to examine touch discrimination, e.g., asking the child to identify an object in a bag using his hands. For children with language problems, pictures of the object may be provided to account for that difficulty. She will also look for signs of sensory discomfort: flinching when touched unexpectedly on their back, reactions to movement etc. She may also ask the child to curl up like a ball, or stand on one leg with eyes closed. These activities provide information about how the child is processing information from the balance receptors (vestibular) as well as those in the muscles and joints (proprioception).

Motor: the OT uses activities and/or standardised tests to assess this broad area of development. While the child is playing or doing certain activities, she observes how the child uses his hands, positions his body, uses his balance or solves something he cannot do (e.g., fitting a puzzle piece). The tasks assess difficulties in balance, body awareness, coordination (bilateral and eye–hand), hand skills, and their impact on practical everyday activities.

Balance is used while moving or maintaining a position. Good balance is required for all motor activities, and especially when the child is using his hands to catch a ball, or draw with a pencil. Bilateral coordination refers to how the child uses the two sides of his body together. As he develops, one hand becomes more dominant and dexterous, while the other hand assists. Bilateral coordination is needed to thread beads, do up buttons and cut with scissors efficiently. Hand skills refer to how he uses his fingers to hold different sized objects: pegs, beads, coins, tiny objects, as well as holding a pencil or scissors. The OT will observe eye–hand coordination with a variety of activities: threading beads, placing pegs, colouring, writing.

An element, known as motor planning, contributes to all these activities. This is the ability to organise and perform unfamiliar tasks. Some children have difficulty learning how to perform many activities such as doing up buttons, forming letters, riding a bike, putting on clothing and the like. The frustration these children feel in learning these simple tasks is similar to that of adults in aerobic classes desperately trying to follow the instructor's movements in the correct sequence! Although the movements themselves are not new, the order in which they are needed is, and it often takes a lot of practice to learn them. This is especially true of children with motor planning difficulties; they take a lot more time to learn some tasks which are very easy for other children. Children with motor planning problems present as being uncoordinated and disorganised, and may also have similar problems with speech and language.

Perception: visual perception is how the brain interprets information gained from the eyes. It develops from moving around in the environment (crawling, climbing) which contributes to the awareness of objects and self, and how they relate to each other.

This forms the basis for the development of constructional activities like building with blocks or writing and drawing, as well as discrimination of shape and size. It is important to note the dependency of sensory, motor and perceptual functioning on each other in the overall development of perception. OTs assess perception using activities such as puzzles and pegboard designs as well as standardised tests.

How can occupational therapy help?

The OT is looking for a pattern in the activities that she has observed. For example, if the child has difficulty cutting with scissors, using a fork and knife together, threading beads and doing buttons, the OT may conclude that he has poor bilateral coordination. Findings from the OT assessment may also have links with problems identified in speech and language. The child who is disorganised in his movement may also have other organisational difficulties with speech or language. For example, many children with speech and language problems are poorly coordinated.

The techniques used to remediate the problems are identified through the assessment. Direct treatment can be provided in a one-to-one situation or group treatment with the OT. If a child does not require direct treatment, programmes are developed by the OT and carried out by others, e.g. teachers, parents. Usually such programmes concern the development of certain skills (e.g. how to dress), or guidelines pertaining to development in general. Advice to parents and teachers or teaching assistants may be provided verbally or through programmes.

OTs may also prescribe aids or devices for the school or home: a 'pencil grip' reminds the child where to hold the pencil and encourages the proper grasp and a 'dycem mat' stabilises paper while writing. It is important to remember that such devices are compensatory techniques. That is, through treatment the child may develop a proper pencil grasp or learn to use his non-dominant hand to assist, instead of relying on such devices. Ideally, it is best if the child uses these devices in conjunction with treatment to help carry over in other situations.

Finally, OTs may also provide advice on positioning. At school the child should be sitting at a proper sized table with his feet firmly touching the ground. Some children may also benefit from doing activities in different positions. For example, the child can lie on his stomach to read or watch television. Painting can also be done while in a 'crawl' position or while kneeling. These positions provide alternative experiences which challenge balance and promote good body awareness.

To best meet the needs of the child, the OT will usually employ one or a combination of approaches. For the young child these will all be based on the medium of play. The aim of intervention is to build his self-esteem by encouraging the development of particular skills.

CHAPTER 5

Labels and Diagnosis
What Happens After Assessment

Once a child has been identified as having a difficulty parents usually want to know precisely what that difficulty is. Friends or family may ask why you are taking your child to the clinic, or why he is having extra help at school. It is often easier to explain if there is a label which can be used that is understood by others. However, as we shall see in the present chapter, applying a label has its own pitfalls.

What use is a label?

The therapist will consider the information obtained through assessment and come to a conclusion about the pattern of strengths and weaknesses in the child's speech, language and related skills. More often than not she will then ascribe a label or diagnosis to the presenting difficulty, and will continue to use this label in written reports and letters which may be widely circulated to parents, carers and other involved professionals. It shold be noted that labels and diagnoses may change over time, as the child changes.

Parents are often rightly concerned about such labels and it is therefore extremely important for the therapist to explain their meaning and purpose. In some instances parents have been concerned about their child for some time and the ascribed label or diagnosis may serve to alleviate some anxiety and justify parental concern. In others there may be resentment and some fear that their child is not being assessed as an individual with a profile of strengths and weaknesses, but is labelled in order to place him in a 'diagnostic category'.

This too can happen when a parent is reluctant or not ready to accept the implications of the label and their child's disability. There will also be occasions when professionals involved with a child choose different labels or have different perceptions of the child's difficulties.

It is understandable that such different views prevail as they often reflect the training, experience and orientation of the professional involved; nevertheless this is not very helpful to the parents. In addition, the severity of the speech and language problem may have resource implications for local authorities whose staff may therefore be reluctant to acknowledge the extent of the difficulty and the educational and financial implications of such an impairment. In some instances parents are effectively being asked to choose which view to believe. This is especially true when one professional maintains that mainstream schooling is appropriate and another is recommending language unit provision. In our experience this position is unhelpful and should be avoided.

In some cases there may be a reluctance to provide a diagnosis at all. This could be for a number of reasons:

1. The impairment is complex and cannot be conveniently fitted into any one diagnostic category.

2. The type of impairment the child has becomes more clearly defined with age. This makes it easier to be sure what is wrong once the child moves beyond the age at which most children are proficient in their language development.

3. There may be additional factors to consider for the child, his family and the therapist if the child's first language is other than, or in addition to, English. In such cases it is sometimes more difficult to ascertain whether or not the difficulty is primarily to do with speech and language acquisition as a skill, regardless of what language that may be, or if the child is simply muddled, switching between two or more languages. This situation is often complicated by lack of appropriate assessment materials for languages other than English, and inadequate specialist interpreting and translation services within the health and education authorities.

4. It is of course possible that the child may have a specific condition which is not necessarily widely recognised by all speech and language therapists, paediatricians or psychologists. In this case the parents should seek a second opinion until they are satisfied.

It is, however, important to recognise that labels and diagnosis do serve some very useful functions. They allow services to acknowledge that there indeed is a recognisable problem and one for which the appropriate provision is necessary. This enables those concerned to identify trends and levels of need and plan resources accordingly. In addition, resources to meet the child's needs may only follow if a recognisable label is used. Labels and diagnosis also allow speech and language therapists to group children together with others who are experiencing parallel difficulties for the purposes of intervention. The benefits of group therapy are many and include opportunities for parents to meet others whose children have similar difficulties.

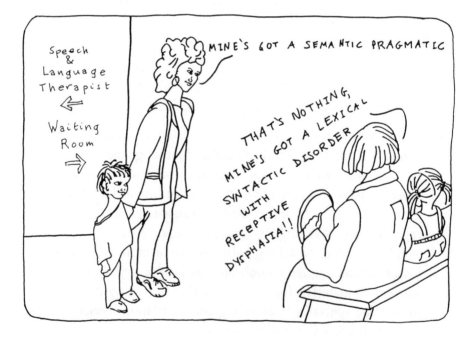

Figure 3

Having looked at the value of labels and diagnosis it is important to bear in mind two points. First, the study of speech and language impairments is still in its infancy and there remains a considerable amount of disagreement among professionals and related literature about exactly where the boundaries between different sub-categories of the conditions fall. The second is the need to make those working with your child accept that there is a problem. This is often more important than the labels themselves. Similarly it is much more important and useful to know exactly what your child can and cannot do, and needs to do next, than to be able to say he has this, or that, condition.

Who uses labels?

There are many labels in common usage. We begin by looking at those used commonly by doctors and go on to consider the way that these children are seen by those involved in providing education.

In subsequent sections we will look at labels used by the speech and language therapist. We will only mention the most common in this chapter, but should parents come across alternative labels they should seek clarification from their speech and language therapist.

Many of the labels used for children with speech and language impairments have their origins in terminology derived from *medicine*. These often suggest a cause for the disorder based on information gathered from studies of adult neurological impairment following some form of brain damage such as a stroke or head injury. Such terms, whilst still in use are not always helpful as they are not shared by colleagues in education who will inevitably work with the children at school. The most widely used examples are *developmental dysphasia/aphasia* and *dyspraxia*. Dyspraxia will be discussed later on when talking about specific disorders. Such terms were, up until the 1970s, also used to describe some similarities between adults and children presenting a similar profile of difficulties.

However, the comparisons are limited. We assume that adults who have suffered a stroke have already developed language skills, and were thus not trying to develop them, but 'find them again'. Children with speech and language difficulties may present at any age but in most cases the skills fail to develop rather than disappear. The terms dysphasia and aphasia also imply that there has been some brain damage or 'lesion', and this is the cause of the problem. This can then be demonstrated by sophisticated diagnostic techniques such as brain monitoring equipment.

The same cannot be said for children. Very rarely is there evidence of this type. The more likely assumption for a child would be that the neurological apparatus is developing more slowly or in an unusual way about which we know very little.

Colleagues in *education* bring an alternative perspective on the child through their different professional training and experience. While some teachers and psychologists may use standardised tests and checklists, more usually they will observe the child at school and make judgements about their performance in relation to other children. It does not necessarily follow that they will relate their information to a 'norm' or 'age equivalent'. More often a teacher will describe a child's abilities and his rate of progress across a range of activities and the key stages of the National Curriculum, and have knowledge about what the child has achieved in relation to those key stages.

Historically, children with special needs have been variously labelled within the education system. Such labels and their use and popularity rise and fall with the prevalent political, economic, social, cultural and educational climate of the time. Educational legislation has encouraged a move away from labels and categories towards description of a child in terms of strengths and difficulties and the provision required to meet their needs. This is much more useful to parents, teachers and other professionals who need to plan for the special educational needs of the child. Whether the child is in a special or a mainstream school, such descriptions help identify what the child can already do and therefore 'needs to do next' in order to make progress.

We have discussed a number of different uses of labels. In *speech and language therapy* a combination of descriptions and labels will be used. We now turn to the labels that speech and language therapists use, and give some examples that you may encounter in reports.

Primary or secondary impairments

The first distinction to be aware of is the differentiation made between *primary* and *secondary* language impairments. 'Primary' language impairments are said to be those where the difficulty is specific to language; hence the term *specific language impairment*. Use of the word 'specific' indicates there are no other major contributory factors such as a significant degree of neurological impairment, hearing loss, emotional and behavioural difficulties or environmental deprivation. Thus, if the child has a language difficulty which cannot be attributed to, or be part of, any of the above, then he must have a problem which is 'specific' to language.

Isolating conditions in this way is known as 'definition by exclusion'. This may be appealing in that it would be difficult to categorise some children other than in this way. However, it should be recognised that the similarities between children in this group may not be great. They may, indeed, all have specific language difficulties but the manifestation of these in the child will in each case be different and have different implications for intervention and learning. Although the nature of this category is the subject of much debate it continues to be used as the justification for provision for such children in language units, or other specialist provision where children whose difficulties with language are said to be specific and not part of a pattern of more general difficulties or secondary to another impairment.

A 'secondary' language impairment is said to be that which results from, or is part of, another condition. For example, a child with Downs Syndrome is very likely to have speech and language difficulties but there is also a wider profile of learning difficulties which also need to be addressed. In addition, children with hearing impairments and cerebral palsy will have speech and language problems which are a consequence of the primary disorder caused by hearing loss or neurological impairment.

We cannot always draw a simple distinction between primary and secondary impairments. It is possible to see a child with a primary difficulty in learning (for example, a child with a general pattern of learning difficulties) who in addition has a specific speech and/or language impairment. While there is some agreement between professionals as to the nature of a specific label or diagnosis, it may be helpful to describe these labels under the following headings. Parents will then be able to better understand why different labels or diagnoses are offered by the various professionals they may meet.

Language delay or language disorder?

Language delay and disorder are labels frequently used by speech and language therapists and other professionals. They are largely generic terms used to describe the process of language development.

'Delay' implies that speech and language is following a normal developmental pattern. These children are often slow to start speaking, but the rate of language development is often similar to that of other children; nevertheless they remain behind their peers unless they are given appropriate help. Indeed, in the very early years some slow starters seem to catch up on their own. This term is often used for pre-school children and it suggests that the child is likely to make up the delay with time and appropriate intervention. Some children who appear to be slow starters get there in the end and are indistinguishable from their peers in school.

This term is also used for children who have general learning difficulties because the child's stage of development is more likely to correspond to that of a younger child. Again, the term tends to be used for the younger child. When the child reaches the age of seven or so, the concept of delay becomes more difficult to apply because most children who are going to catch up spontaneously will have done so. In addition, the speech and language patterns of a seven-year-old are not really comparable to that of a younger child in any meaningful way. His experiences will be quite different from a child of, say, five, and this will be reflected in the vocabulary and syntax used. This label, therefore, tends to become redundant with time.

'Disorder', by contrast, suggests there is an abnormal pattern of speech and/or language development. It is not always clear whether this means that the components of language – phonology, syntax and semantics – or of speech, are out of synchronisation with one another or whether it is the sequence in which skills are learned which is disrupted. If it is the former, many children will fit into this category because a considerable number of them will have relative strengths and weaknesses. Some will have poor phonological skills, others will be very clear when they speak but have difficulty in understanding language or using syntax. If it is the latter, the number of children will be very small because there is very little evidence that children with serious speech and language difficulties who attend language units learn language in a different sequence from other children.

There is also a qualitative dimension to the distinction between these two terms. 'Delay' is considered less severe and less persistent than 'disorder'. Unfortunately, the terms are not easily separated, especially at an early stage in the child's development. There is a tendency, therefore, to use the label 'language delayed' until the age the child should have caught up, and 'disordered' if their difficulties do not resolve. It is very difficult to predict precisely which children will go on to have a speech and language disorder when confronted by a two- or three-year-old. We do know that there are many three-year-olds who are delayed in speech and language development in the first instance, who continue to have those difficulties through into their school years.

However useful these terms may be in 'categorising' speech and language impairments they cannot alone predict the outcome for the child and will probably not be very useful when it comes to helping your child's language development. These terms will, however, give you a common language to discuss your child's difficulty with the range of professionals and other parents you may meet. Both 'delay' and 'disorder' are often further divided into predominantly *receptive* and *expressive* problems. Thus a child may present with normal receptive language, or comprehension, but an expressive delay or disorder. It is very unusual for children to have normal expressive language and delayed comprehension skills, but the reverse is not an uncommon problem. The more common combination is where both receptive language and expressive language are affected to some degree.

Language impairments

Language impairment is an umbrella term covering all conditions in which language skills are significantly different from other areas of development. We will now give an overview of some labels used for language impairments.

Receptive language disorder / receptive dysphasia

This term, whilst widely used by speech and language therapists to imply difficulties in understanding spoken language, gives little information on the severity of the disorder for the child. Where a child is described as having a severe receptive language disorder, further information regarding the child's capacity to understand language will inform others of its impact on the child at home, in the classroom and socially. The term 'receptive dysphasia' is a more specific term but is less widely used. It is largely reserved for children who display extreme difficulties understanding the spoken word. In the absence of wider developmental difficulty the child appears simply to be unable to retain and process spoken language.

Initially, such children may be completely 'tuned-out', isolated and uncommunicative. Additionally, there may be behavioural difficulties caused by the child's inability to understand what is required of him. Social conventions and the rules of interaction may be a mystery to him. These children can be helped by means of specific therapeutic programmes which may include signing. Signs enable the therapist, together with the parents and teachers, to convey meaning using another modality, i.e. a visual channel. For such children meaning comes slowly and it is unlikely that they would cope within a mainstream school environment where both the medium of teaching and social interaction with peers is conducted through spoken language.

Semantic pragmatic disorder

This is a disorder which was first identified by this name in the early 1980s and has since become widely recognised among therapists, specialists and teachers working with specifically language-impaired children. These children are often very slow to develop language and when at three or four they do begin to speak, they are often very repetitive or 'echolalic' – that is, repeating what they have just heard, or repeating that which they have heard some time ago. Often such repetition is inappropriate to the context, meaningless to the listener and not very useful to the child. Such children seem to have grasped that saying something keeps the conversation going, but they seem singularly unable to acquire the rules of social interaction and language use which allow us to take turns and participate fully in the conversation.

When tested using formal assessments of the type identified in Chapter 3, these children show an unusual relationship between their expressive skills and their comprehension. Whereas for many children poor comprehension leads to poor expressive language, the reverse seems to be the case for children with semantic pragmatic disorder. In early years they often do poorly on comprehension tests, but they talk a lot and what they say sounds quite complex. For many of these children their understanding improves as they get older. In particular they seem to learn how to respond to very structured situations, such as language testing. However, they continue to have difficulty integrating their knowledge about the real world. Even more significantly they lag further and further behind their peers in their ability to initiate, maintain, repair and close conversations.

For many, the whole process of interaction provokes extreme anxiety. In order to cope they develop strategies which interrupt the flow of communication. Many cannot give up the initiative in the conversation and will talk at length about their favourite topics – buses, toilet paper, tape recorders, fire engines and the like, but make it quite clear that another can only engage in the conversation on their terms. If you try to divert such children, they will often reassert their control by reintroducing another favourite topic. The conversation then falls apart and all too often the participants are left with the feeling of a failed interaction.

The terms 'semantic' and 'pragmatic' suggest this diagnosis was originally derived to refer to a particular group of language-disordered children. Some of the characteristics of this disorder are also shared by children whose communication difficulties can be said to be on the autistic or social communication disorder continuum. As the word 'continuum' suggests, at the one end there are children who display a significant range of behaviours normally associated with a diagnosis of autism. At the other end are children with less marked autistic features and more successful communication skills. These children share many of the features of autism in its mildest form, but are nevertheless on the continuum. Clearly, semantic pragmatic disorder incorporates aspects of both a language impairment and social communication disorder and will probably remain on the fringes of the two conditions.

This diagnosis can be confusing for parents because there may be some disagreement between professionals about the diagnosis itself. For many parents and professionals the label of semantic pragmatic disorder is more acceptable than that of 'autism' – a term which is frequently perceived as more serious. Parents should in this case ensure that they understand where their child's most profound difficulties lie and are sufficiently guided by professionals in the teaching of strategies which will enable the child to cope.

Lexical syntactic disorder

Like the term semantic pragmatic, lexical syntactic disorder is one which derives from our understanding of linguistic development. Children who have this condition usually present with both comprehension and phonology within normal limits. Their difficulties are confined to the ability to acquire vocabulary and so produce more than the most basic syntactic structures.

Like many language-impaired children, they often appear very quiet in the first instance, and it is often not possible to make an accurate diagnosis until the child becomes actively involved in the process of learning language. It may be clear that they have difficulty acquiring words, and that when words come they are the ones the child has been taught rather than those they have picked up incidentally. In particular, these children acquire a considerable vocabulary of nouns, but have difficulty starting on verbs or other parts of speech. Inevitably this will make it very difficult for the child to move on to using sentences. Indeed, the whole process of acquiring language proves to be a struggle. They may contribute to a classroom activity but often at a minimal level and are unable to express more complex ideas through language.

Such children miss out on the stage of linguistic development where other children automatically assimilate new words together with their meaning and begin to rehearse them straightaway. They need to learn each new dimension of language in a conscious way, in the way that an adult might teach themselves to learn a new language. Many of these children benefit from the structure of language unit provision and eventually do go on to cope well in mainstream schools. Language is not one of their strengths but they develop strategies for coping in conversation.

Speech disorders

We will look at three examples of speech disorders: phonological disorders, dyspraxia and fluency problems.

Phonological disorders

As discussed in Chapter 1, phonology refers to the process by which children acquire the sounds of speech. Our expectations of children change with their age. We are happy with a limited number of sounds from a two-year-old but anticipate that most children will acquire all the sounds of speech with very few exceptions or residual immaturities (e.g. s → th), and use them correctly by the time they start school.

None the less there are some children for whom the process of phonological acquisition seems to lag behind their other skills. Such children may be referred by their parents, health visitor, GP or other agency to speech and language therapy. The problem for the speech and language therapist is to decide whether or not what appears to be a delay should be treated and how intensively. The key features of a phonological disorder are that a number of the child's speech sounds are pronounced incorrectly or not at all. The important point is that the errors are made in a systematic fashion. Often there are whole groups of sounds which may be affected. A common example of a phonological delay is known as 'fronting'. In this process the child consistently uses speech sounds which are made at the front of the mouth when the correct target would have been a sound made at the back of the mouth. Thus, if we take the 'back' sounds /k/ and /g/ these would be 'fronted' to /t/ and /d/.

Example: cake   → tate   Kate → tate

garden → darden   go   → doh

This is normal in the young child but it is more of a problem when the condition exists in a three- or four-year-old, particularly when we know that a number of similar processes are often in operation simultaneously and this can lead to the child being completely unintelligible. If the child experiences frustration at trying to communicate and is impeded by his poor speech, appropriate professional help should be sought.

Delayed or disordered phonological development can have a profound impact on the development of a child's expressive language. These children often recognise that it is better to limit their 'output' to two words in the hope that they will be understood, rather than try and say a sentence most of which the listener will not understand and may ask for repetition.

Similarly, omission of some sounds can make a big difference to what the child means to say. For example, children commonly omit /s/ when they start to learn speech sounds, but as they develop their meaning and they want to refer to more than one item, they need a plural /s/ to mark it. Similarly, they need /s/ to mark verb tenses and auxiliary verbs such as 'is' and 'was'. Frequently, such children dispense with many such forms and retain a rather telegrammatic, staccato quality to their speech.

Dyspraxia

As mentioned previously, this term emanates from a diagnostic category derived from work with adults with a neurological impairment. Despite any evidence for such brain lesions in children this term continues to be used widely. Children may demonstrate features of dyspraxia but some experience more pronounced difficulties. The label dyspraxia is sometimes applied to young children but is more commonly reserved for children with the most persistent and severe speech disorders.

The definition of dyspraxia is the 'inability to produce a voluntary, purposeful movement on command in the absence of muscle damage'. It refers, therefore, to the child's inability to coordinate aspects of tongue, lip and palatal movements effectively in trying to speak. Thus the child may be able to stick out his tongue to lick an ice-cream, but not be able to do so when asked. The speech apparatus or organs of speech and the links with the brain are complex and it is hardly surprising that difficulties of this type arise. Yet the fact that most children learn to speak clearly by the time they are three suggests this is only another developmental hurdle they must negotiate.

For children with dyspraxia, the speech 'programme' seems to have gone awry. In this disorder it is not simply a matter of replacing one sound, or group of sounds, with another. Sometimes dyspraxic children are able to produce a sound in isolation, e.g. /k/, but as soon as they begin to combine the sound with others, e.g. /k/ and /ey/ = key, the system falters. Indeed the longer or more complex the target word or phrase, the more likely things are to go wrong. Furthermore, when they attempt sounds on a number of occasions these children tend to get the sounds wrong in a different way each time. This is particularly pronounced in polysyllabic words where there is a relatively large amount of information to be processed and acted upon simultaneously. For example, the word 'elephant' may be pronounced as 'edifin','efenun', 'efunt' on consecutive attempts. The frequent results of such effortful and often ineffective attempts at communication are frustration and tiredness. Although, for the purposes of the discussion here, we have focused on the speech development of the children concerned, this condition often has wide implications for the child's more general coordination (see Chapter 4).

Dysfluency

Dysfluency, stammering and *stuttering* are terms used to refer to the process by which children, and indeed adults, seem to get stuck on words or sounds when trying to speak. The result is a hesitant, disrupted speech pattern which at its most severe can be completely debilitating for the individual concerned but, for others with a less severe fluency problem, no more that a mild inconvenience.

In the first three to four years of life many children go through a period of 'normal non-fluency' when they seem to get stuck on sounds or may repeat themselves.

For example:

1. 'My, my, my, my mummy said we're going to the park.'

2. 'My mummy said, my mummy said, my mummy said we're going to the park.'

Again, given the complexity of the process of language acquisition this is hardly surprising and we should not automatically assume that such behaviour constitutes a problem. Indeed, most children 'grow out of it'. We cannot, however, be completely confident of predicting which children will improve spontaneously. Thus it is likely that the parents of a child presenting at a speech therapy clinic with such difficulties will not only be given advice and guidance following assessment, but also be regularly monitored to ensure the problem is resolving. It does seem likely though that those children who 'block' or get completely stuck on a specific sound, or sounds, rather than those who merely repeat words or phrases, will go on to have more persistent difficulties. Such speech behaviours are often associated with 'secondary behaviour' such as considerable tension in the body, and the child may develop tics such as slapping the leg or pointing as a means of both distracting the listener and using a 'starter' to overcome the block.

Summary

For some parents labels can be confusing. For others they can be reassuring. The same may, of course, apply to the professionals that use them. As we have shown, in practice, it is often very difficult to draw clear distinctions between one condition and another. Describing children's individual difficulties is often more useful in planning intervention. Nevertheless, there are a number features which are common to these children and it is to these that we turn in the next chapter.

CHAPTER 6

Issues Commonly Associated with Speech and Language Difficulties

This chapter examines three issues which are often troublesome for many parents of children experiencing difficulties in acquiring language. On first recognising the difficulty the reaction may be 'Why does no one else seem to have a child like mine?' The answer is that they do. We begin by looking at what we know about how many children struggle to communicate effectively. Many parents often go on to ask 'Well, will he just grow out of it?' and we examine the evidence that some children do indeed improve spontaneously or may need relatively little help. Often parents start by blaming themselves for their children's difficulties but, on being reassured that this is most unlikely, go on to ask 'What causes it?' The answer to this question is by no means straightforward but a number of associated factors which may help us unravel something of what is going on are discussed below.

How many children experience such difficulties?

In Chapter 5 we looked at how difficult it can be to draw a line between different types of disorder; it can sometimes be just as difficult distinguishing those who do have problems from those who do not. Parents sometimes say 'Well, he's miles behind his older sister when she was his age.' This may be the case but if we look at the boy's older sister and find that her language development was very advanced, the comparison may not be so revealing at least in so far as it tells us whether he has a problem or not. It is probably more useful to make the comparison with other children in the same class at school, although even then we have to be very careful.

As the child moves up through nursery and into school the teachers are, of course, making similar comparisons, although this time with other children in the class and with other children that they, as teachers, have known in the past. If the teacher has been used to a particular group of children this may well affect his or her expectations of others. For example, if he or she has been used to working with more generally disadvantaged children this may result in a lowered expectation of what a child should be doing for his age.

As already indicated in Chapter 3, speech and language therapists attempt to overcome this problem by using standardised tests – which have been developed on a large number of children who have been shown to be representative of the whole population. We can then compare John with all the other children upon whom the test was originally developed and see how he compares. It is these tests which give us 'age equivalent scores' and 'standard' or 'standardised scores' (see Chapter 3 and 4).

There are essentially three ways of finding out how many children are experiencing difficulties:

1. Go around and ask teachers in a given area how many children they are concerned about

2. Do the same but ask parents, or

3. Assess all the children concerned using standardised tests.

While teachers' judgements are interesting, they can often tell us more about the experience of the teacher than the real number of children with problems. Similarly, if we ask parents we will obviously pick out most of the children with more severe problems but there will be a number of children with less pronounced problems, but problems none the less, about whom parents will not express concern and there may well be a number about whom parents are very concerned but who do not have any real difficulties. The standardised test approach is probably the most accurate way of deciding who does or does not have a problem.

In short, no method is completely fool proof. None the less there does seem to be some sort of consensus emerging that we can expect between five and ten per cent of children to have some sort of difficulty with speech and language in the pre-school years.

Within this group of children we also know that expressive language difficulties are probably much more common than those associated with verbal comprehension. However, we need to be clear that many children who appear to be slow to develop their grammatical skills often have less obvious difficulties in their verbal comprehension. Depending on the area that you look at, the number of children with language impairments probably declines somewhat thereafter. This means that in any class of 30 pre-school children we could expect up to three children with language difficulties of one sort or another. Of course this does not mean to say that they will have 'specific language impairment' of the type referred to in Chapter 5, but they will have communication problems none the less and problems which cannot easily be attributed to known causes such as Downs Syndrome or serious hearing loss.

The natural history of language impairment

We then have to address what is known as the 'natural history'. Do the difficulties that these children experience simply resolve spontaneously? Again the issue is not clear cut and depends on what sort of difficulties the children experience. We know that when children who have been in special schools for their speech and language difficulties are followed up many of them continue to have difficulties well into their teens and beyond. However, a number of these children do manage to reintegrate back into mainstream schools and cope perfectly well. But we need to remember that these children were probably experiencing the most serious difficulties in the first place, so it is hardly surprising that they find it so problematic to fit back in to the system. Furthermore, these children often do not go into such schools until some time after they have had some mainstream nursery and school experience. Older children often have more clearly defined strengths and weaknesses and if their speech or language difficulties are especially pronounced there may be ways that they can compensate for their difficulties by making use of their strengths.

It is much more difficult to be clear about the prognosis for pre-school children. They may stand out as having difficulties which make them different from their peers but the exact nature of those difficulties and particularly the causes of those difficulties are often obscure. We have already commented in Chapter 2 that there is a tremendous variation in the way that children develop language under normal circumstances. This makes simple rules such as 'They should have 50 words by 18 months' difficult to apply. Some children who have not yet achieved this milestone by two or even three years of age may be doing just as well in terms of their language development as their peers in nursery and beyond. Doctors and grandparents often reassure worried parents that children will grow out of these difficulties and clearly there may be some truth in what they say. Not all children who have delays at 18 months, or even three years, need extra help and many seem to manage perfectly well. So can we pick out the children that we are looking for?

To a certain extent this process of identifying children with difficulties happens though the system of checks carried out by health visitors and clinic doctors. They use their clinical judgement and attend training sessions organised by speech and language therapists to develop their awareness of relevant issues so that they can make the appropriate decisions. What they are looking at is not simply a measure of the child's vocabulary but incorporates a variety of different dimensions. For example, their assessment includes a measure of the way that parent and child interact. A child who is simply not communicating at three is likely to cause all sorts of frustration for both parent and child. It is important that these frustrations are addressed earlier rather than later. Similarly, they make some assessment of all the different aspects of language discussed in Chapter 2.

We do know that children who experience difficulties in a number of different aspects of their communication – speech, comprehension and so forth – are more likely to experience persistent difficulties and the more the verbal comprehension is affected the more difficult it will be for them to make use of what they hear. Pre-school children who have syntactic difficulties or who have poor vocabularies in the absence of other difficulties may be less likely to have persistent problems. This does not necessarily mean that the parents of such children should not have plenty of opportunity to discuss what they can do to help their child, but such children are likely to be less of a priority than others with more general linguistic difficulties.

We also need to look at skills beyond those of speech and language before we can make the necessary judgement. We know that many of these children have difficulties with skills associated with speech and language but not necessarily connected with these skills in the minds of parents and teachers. Many of these children go on to have trouble learning to read, write and spell. This is not surprising given that language skills must underpin what we are trying to write. Similarly, we must look carefully at the child's behaviour. All too often teachers pick out children for their bad behaviour in class – for example their inability to attend and their difficulty relating to peers. However, when the child in question is assessed, it becomes clear that the child's language skills are low relative to his or her peers. The child's behaviour may be simply an expression of his frustration and be secondary to an underlying language difficulty.

This confusion is probably less likely when it comes to children with speech difficulties because their problems are more obvious and are widely recognised by all who come into contact with the child. Speech is an area which often gives parents considerable cause for concern. As indicated in Chapter 2, children acquire the appropriate sounds of the language slowly and single sounds that are produced incorrectly at three are unlikely to be of great clinical significance unless they have a dramatic effect on the child's ability to make himself understood. Clearly, children develop these speech skills by practising them in conversation. A child who cannot communicate effectively may be tempted not to communicate at all. This needs to be avoided at all costs and, where it is starting to happen, therapists and teachers may focus, in the initial stages of intervention, on encouraging children to regain their confidence to communicate. Children who pronounce all sorts of words in the same way, for example who produce 'deet' for 'sheet', 'feet', 'seat' are likely to be difficult to understand and their progress needs to be monitored. Signs of anxiety on the part of the child or the parent may be sufficient cause for offering help. Again, if these confusions are the only aspects of the child's communication which is affected and the child's speech seems to be changing of its own accord, albeit slowly, there may be little to worry about.

However, in some of these children there is also a history of difficulties associated with the mouth. Feeding may have been effortful as a baby. The child may continue to dribble long after you might expect them to have controlled this. Even at three or four they may continue to experience difficulties noticing food left around the mouth when eating. They may also be clumsy. If these difficulties co-occur with the speech difficulty, improvement is likely to be slow and intervention is clearly indicated.

For most children these issues are fully covered in the pre-school period and therapists have had a chance to observe the child change with time. However, some children do not encounter the services until they reach school and a decision may be necessary as to whether they need help. This decision will be made between the school, usually the child's teacher, the parent, and the speech and language therapist. In such cases the child's performance in the class after a reasonable period of time is the central issue when it comes to considering whether there is a problem in need of further investigation. Whether the primary focus of intervention should be speech or language work depends on a number of factors which have been discussed in Chapter 3. The older the child is and the more wide ranging the difficulties, the more likely it is that those difficulties will not resolve on their own and therefore the more important that they should be tackled in the school and in the home.

To achieve the fullest possible picture we need to be aware of what we know about the antecedents to speech and language difficulties. These are discussed in greater detail below. Care must always be taken to remember that many language-impaired children will have one or more of these factors in common but lack of such associations does not mean that the problem does not exist, merely that we do not have enough information. In the end, what the child is able to do today is what is most important. Supporting information of the type discussed below may be interesting, but it may not affect the way that we offer to intervene.

Here are some examples.

Child No. 1

Molly was 'small for dates' when she was born and from the start it was clear that her development was slow in a number of areas. For example she walked at two years old and was not toilet trained until she was three and a half years old. Her mother reported that her first word was 'poo' at three and she did not start putting words together for another 12 months. She made slow but gradual progress yet remained very delayed relative to her class mates. She remained in mainstream school with support from a learning support teacher and a special needs assistant and advice from other professionals.

Child No. 2

Jack was referred for speech and language therapy at two years of age. His mother was very worried because he had no clear words even though he was trying to communicate. Information from his family indicated that his early development in everything but speech and language was age appropriate as was his hearing. Although it appeared that his difficulties were primarily in the area of expressive language when assessed by the speech and language therapist he was found to have poor attention and listening, and verbal comprehension well below what you would expect for his age. With help, his attention and comprehension improved, although he continued to find it difficult to follow or engage in conversation. His expressive language, when it came, was difficult to understand. Jack went to a language unit at four years of age and made very good progress. He was subsequently integrated back into mainstream school at seven although he continued to need extra support for his reading and writing.

Child No. 3

Aaron was referred to speech and language therapy at two and a half years old by his health visitor. He was very distractible and his language seemed to be very slow in coming. Initially the speech and language therapist worked with the parents and provided them with ideas to help him focus on language. They went out of their way to give him extra attention and this had the desired effect. He settled down and began to listen to what was said to him. Within three months he had made significant progress and within six was barely distinguishable from his peers.

Is it my fault?

If we take a group of children, there may be all sorts of features that they have in common, but it does not mean that those features are causally related. On the one hand, while it would be true to say that both overall knowledge and foot size increase with age, we would not want to say that the two were related causally in any way. On the other hand, the amount of appropriate conversation directed towards a child is likely to be directly related to the child's subsequent language development later on. The difference between the two is that between correlations and causes.

General abilities and hearing

We know that the majority of children who experience marked difficulties in learning to communicate do so because either all their skills are at a relatively low level in the first place or because they have experienced hearing loss. There may be any number of reasons for their having experienced broader developmental difficulties. For example, many such children have language difficulties associated with known genetic conditions such as Fragile X syndrome or Down's Syndrome. In other cases they may be related to specific experiences associated with the birth process such as *anoxia,* in which the child's brain is starved of oxygen. In extreme cases, malnutrition may have had a similar effect. There may also be a genetic history of learning difficulties. The explanations may be fairly clear in some cases. In cases where there is an obvious learning difficulty of which the speech or language impairment is a part, we speak of the language difficulty being 'secondary' to the primary condition (see the discussion in Chapter 5).

Equally, there are known explanations for children who have had language difficulties secondary to hearing loss. We know that hearing difficulties also run in families, but they are more likely to have been the result of specific infections while the foetus was developing. Where there has been damage to the structures of the ear, such as the cochlea or the auditory nerves, the hearing loss is known as *sensori-neural.* More commonly the condition relates to ear infections which clog up the middle ear. This is known as *serous otitis media* or, more popularly, 'glue ear'. These infections may result from colds in the first instance but may then persist when the cold stops.

For some, however, the effects are particularly pronounced, especially when the hearing loss that the child has experienced persists. The role of hearing has already been touched on in Chapters 2 and 3. However, it is worth adding that there may be an interaction between communication skills and hearing loss in children who have relatively mild hearing losses. Thus they may have a relatively slight hearing loss in the first instance. This makes the processing of what others are saying difficult and, in turn, can result in unclear speech because the child is unsure as to exactly what he has heard. The child's listening skills develop in rather an erratic way. Sometimes they can hear efficiently, but at other times they have to watch faces closely to understand what is being said or turn the television up to hear it. It is hardly surprising in such circumstances that even when the infection has cleared up they may not be able to discriminate spoken language very well when either they or others are speaking. In such cases we might speak of a primary hearing difficulty leading to a secondary difficulty in speech and/or language.

As discussed in Chapters 3 and 5, once we have excluded such secondary speech and language difficulties we are still left with a considerable number of children whose difficulties do not have obvious explanations. What explanations might there be for these primary language difficulties?

Genetic factors

An area which has attracted considerable attention recently is the effect that the child's genetic make up can have on their rate of language development. At an obvious level it would be no surprise if there was as much of a relationship here as for other aspects of behaviour which are inherited. Indeed we know that a great many children who experience language difficulties come from families in which one or either parent had a similar difficulty. Of course, it is not always easy to monitor this because we simply do not know enough about the experience of many parents when they were children. We can ask very general questions such as 'Do you remember having difficulties speaking?' or 'Did you have difficulties reading and writing?', but we cannot be sure that we are looking at the same behaviour as that observed in the next generation. Only one generation back there was little recognition of such difficulties and, except for children with the most extreme difficulties, no educational provision was available. There has been one study which has attempted to show a clear link between difficulties producing specific types of speech sounds across three generations but the exact nature of the relationship remains uncertain and of great technical interest to those concerned with plotting gene maps. In reality, it is extremely unlikely that it will simply be a matter of finding a single gene as it might be for the most obviously circumscribed medical conditions. We are more likely to be speaking of an interrelationship between either a combination of genes or between the genetic make up and the environment.

Medical complications

The most common 'medical' condition which is likely to precipitate language learning difficulties is hearing loss. But since we have dealt with this already we will turn to some others.

If we look for evidence in the birth history we find that many of these children have complex histories. Perhaps they were what is known as 'small for dates', that is, weighing much less than would be expected for their gestational age? Perhaps they were simply very small or born very early? Unusual deliveries are commonly reported as is jaundice and other treatable medical conditions after birth. Many children have experienced periods in intensive care immediately after the birth. Can we then say that these experiences caused speech and language problems? The answer is that although they may be common for the children subsequently picked out with difficulties, these experiences are often associated with generally delayed development and so cannot very easily be said to have a specific relationship to language or speech development. Equally, a considerable number of such children do not have a history of such complications. So even if there is some truth in that these experiences may hold some children back, the same is by no means true for many of those who go on to have difficulties.

There is one association which does need to be taken seriously. Many of the children who have experienced medical complications in the first few weeks of life are at risk of having speech and language difficulties especially if they were sleepy, passive babies. It is often very difficult to communicate effectively with them because they make so few demands. This can lead to feeding difficulties and often leads to frustration. Parents, and especially mothers, can get very upset trying to make their baby feed when they do not seem to want to. This may make communication unrewarding in those first few months and, as we have seen in Chapter 2, it is those first few months which serve as the earliest building blocks of communication development. It is important to recognise that this is not necessarily the case and we must not assume that it has happened in this way, but medical complications may act as a predisposing factor rather than a cause of difficulties.

The most convincing evidence for medical causation comes from conditions in which we know that the child has experienced specific brain damage as a result of damage to the speech and language areas of the brain. These areas are relatively small and such damage must be very localised. In some cases there is evidence of special difficulties with speech or language as a result of general infections of the brain such as meningitis or as a result of trauma such as road traffic accidents. However, in such cases the evidence usually suggests that language is only one of many skills affected. There is a very rare condition in which children experience epilepsy which damages the speech and language areas. This is known as 'temporal lobe epilepsy' after the area where the damage occurs, the area commonly associated with the processing of language. Such damage can result in very severe language difficulties and is sometimes referred to as Landau Kleffner Syndrome.

Social factors

Parents understandably feel responsible for difficulties that their children experience. However, very few people would suggest that parents can be said to be directly responsible for their child's difficulties. The relationship between how we bring up our children and the way in which they learn language is much more complex than a simple relationship between what goes in and what comes out. Although, as we have seen, language is triggered neurologically at the end of the first year of life, inevitably we play a part in encouraging children who seem to want to communicate. People say 'No wonder she speaks the way that she does. Just look at her parents!' If children are regularly exposed to language and have it drawn to their attention, they usually learn to use it quickly and efficiently. There is some variability here, as we have already discussed, but such differences are usually resolved in the first three or four years of life. Children may end up with different styles of interaction, but they can all communicate more or less efficiently. Is there a case then for saying that just as language can be promoted by the input from the parents, it can be effectively slowed down for the same reason?

As we saw in Chapter 2, and as we shall discuss further in Chapter 8 when we discuss particular approaches to intervention, the evidence, such as it is, suggests that children pick up language by having their attention drawn to it in the right context. We do not teach them the grammatical constructions as such. They merely hear them and begin to make the connections themselves. If we do not draw the surrounding world to their attention, does it necessarily have an adverse effect on their speech and language development?

Unfortunately there are a lot of ill-founded assumptions concerning this issue. Too little allowance is often made for the fact that parents interact with their children differently and that difference is not necessarily indicative of a problem. In the past there was a tendency for middle-class professionals to assume that their model of interaction was the right one and parents who were quieter or less obviously interacting were somehow not doing as much for their child as they should be.

However, having said that, we do know that some children's development has been severely retarded because no attempt at all has been made to communicate with them for very long periods in the child's early development. Fortunately this remains relatively rare and is well outside the range of normal parental behaviour. We should not confuse this with more low key but none the less sensitive parents who interact effectively but simply less often than others.

In the end, the most important aspect of early communication is the need to be there for the child when she wants to communicate and to provide as much stimulation as she needs. It is worth reminding ourselves here that stimulation *per se* is not the answer. If the stimulus is too loud or at an inappropriate level, children simply stop listening to it. Children need quiet periods of consolidation as much as they do noisy stimulating activities. It is for this reason that the parent would be wrong to assume that, by simply leaving a television on when the child is in the room, he or she is helping the child. Many young children simply cannot cope with the noise from the television and tune out. Once they do so, of course, it makes it very difficult for them to tune in to other more interesting stimuli because of the background noise. Other children do watch the television almost as if they are in a trance, showing no understanding of what they are watching and seem to have become fixated on the moving colours on the screen. The point is not that television is a bad thing. It needs to be used appropriately so that children feel that they are sharing what is on the screen with others. In itself it cannot promote interaction but watched with another more experienced speaker it can become a valuable conversation piece.

The same is true of much early interaction with children. It is often not a matter of *what we say* in the sense that we do not need to teach the young child in any active sense, but it is the *way that we say it* that is important. The child needs to grow up understanding that she has a role to play in interaction and that what she says is valued by those around her and is useful to her. When parents are placed in circumstances where they find it difficult to provide this sort of support, the child's communication may be affected. The most obvious cause of difficulty for a parent is extreme stress. We all know that no matter how patient we are, there will be times when children infuriate us and there may be times when we need to withdraw to deal with something important, even if that means ignoring the child for a short period. But for some families this becomes a vicious circle. Personal problems or difficulties keeping up with the requirements of everyday life may make it very difficult for the parent to be available for their child and if this goes on for long periods it may have an adverse effect on the child.

Yet we have to remember that most children do learn to communicate perfectly well and most parents would probably admit that they did not do what they know to be right all the time. We have said above that many children with language impairments simply do not interact very effectively themselves. They find it difficult tuning into language and cannot make themselves easily understood. Such children place considerable demands on their parents. It is almost as if their parents have to become 'super parents' picking up nuances of their intended communication and acting as an interpreter for the child so that others can understand what he means. Many parents who experience stress and cannot find enough space for their child alongside their other worries are simply not able to take on the special nature of this task of interpreter. The point is not that stress creates the problem in most cases, simply that it may well make the child's difficulties worse.

Whether parental stress of the type referred to here has the same effect whenever it occurs in the child's development is unclear. Obviously any negative effect on the relationship between parent and child may well have consequences. But that is not the same as saying that it will affect the child's communication development. It seems probable that the real difficulties from the point of view of speech and language occur if the child experiences this in the first three years of life. It is these early years that are of paramount importance for speech and language development as we saw in Chapter 2.

Secondary factors

If we move away now from more obvious causal factors, it is important to consider further associated factors which cannot be said to cause the problems but which come to be so closely associated with them that it may be difficult to disentangle the two. Many children who experience difficulties communicating show their frustration through outbursts of temper. For the pre-school child these may be in the form of aggression towards others or himself. The behaviours may range from tantrums and banging his head against a wall to, more commonly withdrawing from communication. These behaviours are, in many ways, not so very different from the type which we see in younger children – especially during – the 'terrible twos' – that period between the ages of two and three when parents complain that children will do nothing that they are asked. However, whereas these behaviours decline in frequency for most children, they can persist for the language-impaired child.

In many ways the child's frustration is a function of the rising expectation of others. As nursery staff and teachers come to expect certain behaviours from the children in their care, the language-impaired child comes to appear increasingly immature. It is not necessarily that they are regressing back to an earlier set of the behaviours, although this may be the case. It is more likely that their peers in class, having consolidated their linguistic skills, are moving forwards socially at a tremendous rate. Teachers may become frustrated themselves because they do not know how best to handle the child – whether to scold or cajole – and a cycle is set up whereby the child sees himself reflected in the low expectations of others. It is important to recognise that this means his peers as well as his teachers and the other adults around him. Children expect their friends to interact as effectively as they do. Other children may not necessarily be aware what is going wrong when a child in their class does not communicate very effectively. They may comment that he 'doesn't speak properly', but generally they are simply aware of a difference. For many children, especially those in their early years in primary school, difference is all important in defining who you are. Research has shown that children quickly come to treat language-impaired children differently from their other peers.

At this point it is worth picking up a point that will be developed further in Chapters 7 and 10. The current philosophy of integration gives parents, in consultation with professionals, the right to choose to keep their children in mainstream schooling if their needs can be met. The reasons for this are self-evident in so far as this provides an essentially 'normal' environment for the child. However, as we have seen, the experience of the child concerned may be far from normal and this places the onus fairly and squarely on the school to ensure that the child's experience of school is not disadvantageous.

As the child moves through primary school and on into secondary school the obvious negative behaviours may diminish but the child may still be left with a feeling of social vulnerability. It may be difficult to hold a conversation, to understand jokes except when they are very literal or to understand the intended meaning of others. This may continue to single the child out as being different and although he may or may not be teased for it, he is likely to be extremely aware of his difficulties. This often leads to a reluctance to initiate conversation except with familiar people and an inability to be assertive in social situations. For some children this can become the focus of their existence and can lead to depression later on. This is not, of course, true for all children. Those who are more confident and less worried about the response of others are more likely to manage socially.

Finally, we turn to one of the most salient bench marks of the child's school experience, notably the ability to read and write. We know from follow-up studies that children who have difficulties learning to speak and to use language at three often go on to have difficulty with their literacy skills. But what is it about those literacy skills that they find difficult? Studies seem to suggest that children with general language difficulties affecting expressive language and verbal comprehension are the most at risk. Children with these difficulties are often struggling with their language skills at a time when they are being expected to translate those skills into another abstract code – the written form. It is difficult enough for them to code the relationship between the world that they perceive and the words used to describe that world without having to then transfer that world on to paper. Reading works the same way in reverse. They have to be able to decode someone else's intended meaning from the written word. If they struggle to understand when someone is talking about something that they can see, how much more difficult is their capacity to process information from the page?

The relationship between speech development and reading is more complex. Intuitively, it makes sense to say that if the child cannot produce the sound correctly he will not be able to perceive it correctly in the written word. However, for the majority of children with phonological difficulties, this is not necessarily the case. For most of these children their speech difficulties have resolved by the time they begin to develop their reading skills and they seem able to manage the written word without too much difficulty. The exception to this seems to be children who have very severe speech difficulties, especially those of a dyspraxic nature. These children often continue to have literacy difficulties for many years.

Summary

Apart from children whom we know to have language impairments secondary to other conditions such as general learning difficulties and hearing loss, we have to face the fact that we often do not know the cause of the difficulties that the children experience. This is likely to be extremely frustrating for the parents of the children concerned but it is a fact that therapists and parents have to learn to live with. In most cases there is a complex interrelationship between predisposing factors and the environment in which the child develops. It is impossible to be categorical about the relationship because, in the end, each child will respond differently to a different set of circumstances. Nevertheless, there is now a broad consensus that these children are constitutionally predisposed to experience these difficulties.

In the final analysis, the causes are probably less important than how we provide the optimum environment to maximise the child's potential. While the causes and correlations described above may inform our decisions as to what help should be offered, it is important not to dwell on the child's history. To do so is to use the past to determine the future. The most important question is not what caused the difficulties, but what we can do about it. In the coming chapters we examine the educational system in the UK and the way in which it provides for language-impaired children. We then go on to look at specific interventions before considering the role played by the independent sector in providing services for these children and their parents. Finally, we look at the legal implications for parents who are worried that their child is not receiving sufficient help.

CHAPTER 7

What Can We Do About It?
Educational Provision

Provision for children with speech and language impairments, along with other health and educational provision, has been subject to trends and external influences. The prevailing political, economic, social, educational and cultural climate largely dictates where money is spent, and on whom. The 1944 Education Act introduced, for the first time in the UK, education for all and it was the 1970 Education Act that recognised the right to education for all those with special educational needs. This legislation brought children with even the most severe learning difficulties under the remit of the education service, and segregated special education in the form of a range of 'special schools' was developed.

Historically, many children with speech and language disorders were educated in a variety of special schools; the majority being 'delicate' or schools for 'children with moderate learning difficulties'. Indeed, such schools in the absence of more appropriate provision provided, at least in some measure, for the children's needs. Further legislation in the form of the 1981 Education Act provided the first Act specifically concerned with special needs. It was implemented in 1983. Many of the parents reading this will have a child who has a 'statement'. The 1981 Act, the 1993 Education Act and the 1994 Code of Practice relating to special needs will be outlined in the present chapter and discussed in greater detail in Chapter 10. The stages of assessment relating to the Code of Practice and a copy of the Statement of Special Educational Needs can be found at the back of the book.

The 1981 Act, and subsequently the 1993 Act, embodied into legislation the principles of the earlier Warnock Report. This report provided the impetus for the Act, the key elements of which were to recommend:

1. A move away from categories of handicap to description of a child's special educational needs in terms of a continuum of need.

2. A move away from segregation towards integration.

3. The process known as formal assessment leading to the issue of a statement of special educational need.

The Act defines children with special educational needs as those who require additional or different provision from that made generally available within the Local Education Authority. Nationally it was expected that approximately 20 per cent of children may have a special need, or needs, of one type or another at any one point in time during their school career. There was also a suggestion that not more than two per cent of these children would experience more severe and intractable difficulties requiring additional resources over and above those deployed normally within a mainstream school. Most speech- and language-impaired children will already have been identified as having special educational needs before starting school and NHS staff have a 'duty' to inform the Local Education Authority of this identification.

Where a child has already started school and not previously been identified as having special needs, schools will use the framework described in the 1994 Code of Practice to help the child. The child's progress will be assessed and reviewed by the class teacher. Over time the teacher will build up a picture of strengths and weaknesses. If there are concerns about a child's progress and it is felt that the child's needs are not being met within what is normally available a teacher may decide the child has special educational needs and schools, by law, have to publish a policy on their action and reponses to special needs and have to take heed of the Code of Practice. Schools have a duty to involve parents in all stages of any special needs intervention and for a child with a speech and language difficulty they may, with the consent of the parents seek advice from other professionals outside the school. This may, in the first instance be a speech and language therapist, educational psychologist or an advisory teacher from the support services.

It is important to understand that some special needs can be identified and addressed within the first three stages of the Code of Practice and that a move to stage four where the Local Educational Authority consider the need for a statutory assessment may be unnecessary.

However, where the LEA believe a child appears to require different or additional provision from that already made available. they will consider the need for a statutory assessment and if appropriate ask for a multi-disciplinary assessment which may lead to the issuing of a statement of special educational need. Indeed, such a request can be made by parents direct to the Local Education Authority. The assessment consists of a request by the Local Education Authority to parents and all those involved with the child, to submit what is known as 'Advice'. This is, in effect, a written report. When all the 'Advice' has been received, an 'officer' of the Local Education Authority, normally a statementing officer and/or educational psychologist, will consider all the Advice and decide whether to draw up a proposed statement. The LEA can, at this stage decide not to issue a statement.

The proposed statement will be distributed to parents and all those professionals who have submitted Advice. If the proposal is agreed, the statement will be finalised. There are many different statementing 'styles' with one education service writing quite different statements from another. One source of continued heated debate is the inclusion of speech and language therapy under 'educational' or 'non-educational' provision. Much has been made of the Lancashire Judgement (1989) when it was adjudged at a tribunal that except in rare cases, speech and language therapy should be considered educational provision. In practice, however, this is only case law and not legislation, and many speech and language therapists have had, and continue to have, difficulty in persuading the local authority to follow this example.

This impasse is the result of reluctance on the part of both health authorities and local authorities to accept responsibility for the provision of speech and language therapy to statemented children. The 1994 Code of Practice has failed to clarify this issue, placing *prime* responsibility for provision at the door of the health authority, but *ultimate* responsibility for ensuring provision is made rests with the education service. This controversy is not local, but continues at a high level and it will take new government initiatives to change the status quo. Collaborative responsibility for planning and resourcing would seem to be the way forward but with no legal context this remains ambiguous. The 1993 Education Act and 1994 Code of Practice have further implications for the speech- and language-impaired child. The Code of Practice is not legally binding as it is not part of the 1993 Act. Essentially the Code is written guidance to which health authorities and LEAs 'must have regard'. There are however legal obligations which became statutory in September 1995.

Those parts of the Code which are particularly relevant to children with speech and language impairments are the stages of assessment which may lead to a statutory responsibility for initiation of a formal assessment and changes in the timescale for statementing and the annual review process.

There is now a much tighter timetable for completion of the statement and the 'proposed statement' (previously known as the 'Draft') must also state different institutions which would meet the child's special educational needs. The completed statement must be achieved within 26 weeks of the proposal to make an assessment and parents can name their preferred school. In reality, lack of capital expenditure may mean there are few options available, thus limiting parental choice.

Pre-school children and community clinics

As described earlier, the first point of contact for parents with the speech and language therapist is likely to have been a community or local clinic, or Child Development Centre. It is again likely that intervention or provision for the child will take place in one or other of these two venues if the child is very young and not attending school or nursery. There is wide variation nationally on the range of provision of services to these children, and on the methods of service delivery.

Initially a therapy programme will be drawn up by the speech and language therapist in consultation with the parents and in consideration of other information relevant to the child's functioning gained from the assessment by other professionals. Targets or goals for the child will be identified and worked towards by the therapist and parent, and progress regularly reviewed and evaluated. Children may also be offered blocks of therapy for set periods and then allowed a period without direct intervention to consolidate the new skills learned. Such intervention may be on an individual and/or group basis depending upon the needs of the individual child and his ability to cope in a group.

Many therapists working with children with severe speech and language impairments recognise that clinic-based therapy will, as the child gets older, be inadequate to meet the child's needs.

While some of the foundations for the learning of language can be laid down at this time, it is often clear that the child will require further intensive specialist intervention that is not available in most community clinics. This time, however, is often very useful for parents in that it offers opportunities for discussion with the therapist and observation of the child within a controlled and confidential setting.

Language units, classes and groups

Where the child's difficulties have not been resolved with clinic-based therapy, or in-school supprt and appear to be specific and longer term, placement in a language unit or language class may be recommended. Clinic-based therapy is generally inappropriate for children with severe difficulties who are attending mainstream school. The availability, location, access and type of provision available in such units varies enormously.

Language units in various forms can be found in community clinics, social services Under Fives Centres and nurseries. They may also be found attached to mainstream primary schools. Infrequently they are found in secondary schools. They are also found within, or on the same site as, special schools catering for a range of special educational needs. There are also specialist independent schools catering for children with speech and language difficulties.

Access to such units again varies considerably. Those sited within clinics and social services facilities are usually for the young pre-school child and would not require the child to have a 'statement' in order for admission to be considered. Placement in such units is usually at the discretion of the parents and the local speech and language therapy service and the education services may not be involved at all, if the child is not attending a nursery school or of statutory school age. Many units sited within educational facilities, however, do require children to have statements, or at least for the statutory assessment process to have been initiated. There is often considerable pressure for places in such units, with the numbers of children requiring such provision far outstripping the supply. As a consequence of this demand and the move towards integration of children with special needs, many children who might previously have attended language units will instead be 'supported in mainstream'. Selection of children for placement will vary according to local priorities and resources and in consideration of the child's individual needs and the alternative facilities available to meet them.

Different types of language units

There is a wide variety in the type of provision within language units and we will describe those most commonly available.

Community clinic units/groups and social services day nursery/ under fives facilities

Many of these units were set up by speech and language therapists in the absence of provision within the education authority. These units cater for pre-school children and may be full or part-time provision. Some are staffed solely by speech and language therapists and nursery nurses/assistants and some may have teacher input. There are usually fairly prescriptive entry and exit criteria which are largely based on exclusion of 'other' factors. For example: 'no child with a primary hearing impairment', 'children whose non-verbal skills appear to be within, or potentially within, normal limits' etc. These criteria are meant to ensure some degree of homogeneity within the group selected and often exclude children whose difficulties are not specific to speech and language (see discussion on specific language impairment in Chapter 5).

Children whose speech and language difficulties continue to require intensive intervention following a period at such a unit have a number of alternatives for future placement.

Language units attached to mainstream primary school

This type of specialist provision has grown since the late 1970s. They aim to offer a 'broad and balanced' curriculum which takes into account the child's primary difficulties with speech and language. Thus the curriculum is delivered in such a way that it is accessible to this group of children. For example, National Curriculum targets will be broken down into clearly defined stages of learning. Teaching targets will be presented in a variety of different ways with emphasis on visual presentation, rehearsal and repetition of materials. The child's strengths will be used to facilitate learning. A signing system such as *Makaton* or *Paget–Gorman* may also be used to add another dimension through which the child can learn. Classes are small in size (8–12 children) and curriculum planning is undertaken jointly by teachers and speech and language therapists. Teachers in language units may have no specialist training in speech and language disorders, but experience in working with this group of children and collaboration with speech and language therapists often results in the development of considerable expertise which would generally not be found in a mainstream classroom. Some language unit and mainstream support teachers may have undertaken further studies in this field.

Children attending these language units may attend on a full- or part-time basis depending upon local policies, procedures and resources. An individual education programme will usually be drawn up for each child with joint teaching/therapy aims which are monitored, evaluated and regularly reviewed. Children will receive whole class, small group and individual teaching/therapy depending upon their needs and learning style. Some children attending language units may have behavioural difficulties as a result of their language impairment. Staff within the unit will invariably have a level of expertise in managing these problems. Often when the child realises he is in an environment in which he can at last understand what is required and participate in activities at his own level, such unwanted behaviour decreases. At the same time, strategies used by the therapists and teachers to enable the child to participate will enhance the child's opportunities for successful communication. With this type of appropriate help the child will then develop his own coping strategies and grow in confidence and self-esteem. This, in turn, will enable the child to make more rewarding social relationships with peers and adults alike.

Most language units today also offer integration into the mainstream school for children when they are able to benefit from this experience. Generally, assembly, singing and music are whole-school activities and unit children will be expected to participate. As the child progresses with his speech and language development and curricular skills, an integration programme will be drawn up by the unit staff and mainstream class teacher. Initially, the child may integrate for one activity or subject only, with the unit therapist or teacher accompanying him to facilitate a successful integration experience; the level of integration will be increased when the child is able to cope with the increased demands of a mainstream classroom and is less dependent upon the presence of the speech and language therapist, class teacher or assistant.

Pros and cons of language unit provision

It would seem that there has always been a debate among professionals and parents about the placement of children in language units. It must be said that there is little in the way of substantial research to show that children attending language units 'do better' than those who do not. This would appear to be largely a consequence of lack of any research rather than failure to prove their efficacy. Certainly there is local and anecdotal evidence to support language unit provision with many units returning children to mainstream education significantly more able to cope. This would appear to be particularly true where appropriate intervention such as a language unit was initially available at a pre-school age.

One of the main areas of contention often raised by professionals within education is that children attending language units are isolated from their 'normal' peers and not exposed to 'a language-rich environment' or 'normal models of language' from other children. However, the vast majority of children with specific speech and language difficulties have already been exposed to such 'normal models' both at home and at school, but clearly to little effect as they continue to present with severe speech and language difficulties. The 'language-rich environment' is often inappropriate for speech- and language impaired children where verbal information needs to be broken down into understandable chunks and the language environment controlled. An 'overload' of language and activity in a busy mainstream classroom may only serve to confuse the child further and result in isolation or frustration.

An irrefutable disadvantage of placement in a language unit is that the child will not be at the same school as siblings or other children who are members of his local community and will be bussed to the unit. This could potentially limit his access to shared local community activities, play opportunities, the social relationships that may develop as a result, and the feeling of belonging to the community. Many language units also only provide for children in the infant age range, that is up to seven years. Children with severe speech and language impairments may require further specialist provision that is not locally available after this age, and in reality parents are left with the choice of residential school or mainstream.

A further issue to be considered with placement in a language unit is the child's eventual return to the local mainstream school. Schools are no longer obliged to hold places, even where this is the local neighbourhood school, for children who come from alternative provision. In practice, a secured place depends to some degree on the popularity of the school and the number of places available, siblings who may already be on roll, the attitude of the headteacher to children with special needs, and the level of in-school support offered following the child's transfer.

However, despite the disadvantages noted above, children with specific speech and language disorders largely fail to benefit sufficiently from an unsupported mainstream placement. Poor attention, listening skills, difficulty in understanding and using language and often poorly developed social interaction skills ill-equip this group of children for the demands of the classroom. Spoken language is the main medium for teaching and the ability to attend, listen, understand and communicate in a group are fundamental to 'meaningful access' to a broad and balanced curriculum, and the development of successful peer relationships. Ultimately, it is for parents to weigh up the pros and cons of this specialist provision in the light of their knowledge of the child and the information received from professionals working with them.

Mainstream school with support

The 1981 Act asserted the right of children with special educational needs to be educated as far as possible in ordinary schools. It remains a challenge for all schools to extend their flexibility so as to respond to pupils' learning needs. Data received by the Department for Education showed that between 1982 and 1987 there was an overall drop from 1.53 per cent to 1.41 per cent in the percentage of pupils aged 5–15 years in special schools in England. This study also revealed wide variations between different Local Education Authorities with some showing significant increases.

Funding for children with special educational needs within mainstream schools has been profoundly affected by government legislation. The 1988 Education Reform Act made barely any reference to how special needs education was to be maintained or furthered. Funding for schools largely depends on the number of their pupils, and secondary schools compete for pupils through their position in league tables of aggregate achievement in the National Curriculum. Both of these elements may constitute a possible disincentive for schools to admit children with special needs and to allocate resources to support them. At the same time Local

Education Authorities were required to delegate increasing proportions of their funds to schools, thus reducing the amount of funds held centrally to support special needs children. There is a considerable body of anecdotal evidence suggesting that both ordinary and special schools are finding it difficult to meet pupils' special educational needs. The trend is reflected in increases in the percentage of children with statements of special needs in Local Education Authorities. If schools cannot fund the resources they need to meet pupils' needs, the statementing procedure offers a way of obtaining additional resources from the Local Education Authority.

Thus children with speech and language difficulties attending mainstream schools may receive hugely varying levels of support and intervention depending upon the Local Education Authority in which they live, and whether or not they are the subject of a statement. Speech and language therapy services to children in mainstream schools also vary widely. Some NHS Trusts have provided funds for therapists to work with these children and others have not. Joint funding initiatives between health and education have also been forthcoming in some areas. In others, where the NHS has failed to provide sufficient resources, the education authority has funded posts. There continue to be many areas of the country where there is no integrated school-based service for these children. Meeting the speech and language needs of children with specific difficulties within the mainstream is a relatively new initiative. As such, many different models of 'service delivery' have been developed and it is only over time and with evaluation that we will be able to see which models are most effective and those which in economic terms reflect 'value for money'.

Generally speaking, the speech and language therapist will liaise closely with all those involved with the child. This will include parents, class teachers, the schools' special needs coordinator (a school post required by the 1994 Code of Practice), the local learning support service and the educational psychologist. Programmes will be drawn up by the relevant professionals and teaching/therapy targets set. These targets will be regularly evaluated and reviewed and the programme updated accordingly. The child may have individual or small group sessions within the mainstream classroom or resource base, carried out by a speech and language therapist alone or more usually together with a learning support teacher and/or special needs assistant. The level and frequency of therapy

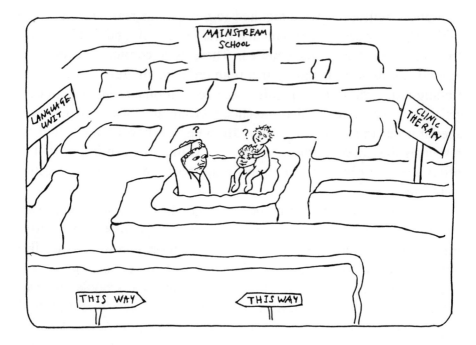

Figure 4

will depend upon the child's individual special needs and the resources available to meet them.

The essence of successful intervention within mainstream is collaboration between the speech and language therapist and those staff working regularly with the child. Time must be allowed for training, joint assessments and planning if the programme is to be successful.

Pros and cons of mainstream provision

It is difficult to assess the relative advantages or disadvantages of mainstream placement for a child with specific speech and language difficulties. Generally, for children with severe impairments, a great deal of individual and small group work would be required to even begin to meet their needs. In practice, such resources are rarely available and the child may indeed make some progress in his infant/primary school years. It is important to distinguish here between academic and social progress. It is often the transition to junior school with greatly increased demands in the classroom that make the true nature of the child's difficulties clear to his teachers.

Many specifically speech and language impaired children have some difficulty acquiring literacy skills and this adds another dimension to the resourcing issue. The attractions of mainstream education for parents are many. The child may be less 'stigmatised' as he is not attending a special school or unit. He will be at school with his neighbours and belong to a local community. He will be offered a 'broad and balanced curriculum' which may not be so easy to deliver in alternative provision, and he will have appropriate models of behaviour and social interaction from which he may learn.

Ultimately, it is for parents to choose which provision best suits their child. It is important for parents to ensure that the provision made within a mainstream school is enough not just to 'maintain' or 'contain' the child, but to enable him to progress educationally, socially and emotionally. The review process held by the school is the opportunity for parents to find out how well their child is progressing and what needs to be done next.

Local authority special school provision

As mentioned earlier, in the past, children with speech and language difficulties were often educated in schools for children with learning difficulties or 'delicate' schools. Many of the latter continue to take children with a range of complex special educational needs, from chronic asthma to autism. Many such schools have teachers and assistants experienced in working with children with a range of special needs. They have expertise in differentiating the curriculum (breaking it down into smaller, more easily accessible components), and in devising individual learning programmes for children. They also often have considerable skill in managing difficult behaviour.

However, the move towards integration has to some extent changed the range of special needs found in special schools. It is often children with the most complex and profound special needs who are placed here in their primary years. These children may not provide an appropriate peer group for the speech and language-impaired child, either socially or educationally. Children with more general learning difficulties attending special school are likely to have a slower rate of learning than others and there may not be the opportunity for the non-verbally able language impaired child to reach his or her full potential.

Children leaving primary age language units where it is clear that they will not cope with mainstream secondary school, and where there is no secondary language unit, may be placed in these schools. It is probably true to say that if by this age the child continues to have difficulties which preclude him from accessing the curriculum in any meaningful way in mainstream, then appropriate specialist provision may be in the child's best interests.

Independent special school provision

There are a number of special schools, both day and residential for children with specific speech and language disorders (see Chapter 9). In practice, local authorities will be reluctant to seek a place for a child at such a school as the costs involved are very substantial indeed when compared with local provision. These schools are usually very well staffed with teachers and assistants experienced in working with speech and language impaired children and a considerable number of specialist speech and language therapists. Classes are small, resources are often impressive and the whole curriculum is planned with the child's difficulties in mind. There are opportunities in such schools for specifically speech and language impaired children to develop their strengths and talents while at the same time receiving considerable help for their difficulties. The disadvantages of a residential placement are obvious, and in order to attend as a day pupil families may have to re-locate to be near enough to the school. These independent schools do, however, provide for the minority of children whose needs may be less adequately met elsewhere.

Summary

Over the last 50 years the needs of children with speech and language difficulties have come to be recognised. However, the services available to them often depend upon a variety of factors, not least of which is the area in which the family lives. Parents should make a point of finding out what is available and of making sure that the help that their child is receiving matches their child's needs. One of the greatest difficulties from a parent's perspective is knowing what your child *does* need. Often you are aware that your son or daughter is not doing as well as they might, but find it harder to pinpoint what sort of help should be offered. Many parents simply do not know what speech and language therapists do and cannot, therefore, make an informed decision as to whether that is what is needed. In the next chapter we turn to ways in which speech and language therapists work with children.

CHAPTER 8

What Can We Do About It?
Different Approaches to Intervention

Once we have recognised that a child has delayed language development the next question that we must address is how best to go about helping him improve his communication skills. This chapter discusses this issue. It begins with a discussion of the aims of therapy and goes on to look at some of the practical considerations that need to be made when planning therapy. We consider the advantages and disadvantages of group versus individual treatment. A number of specific approaches to therapy/treatment are then introduced alongside reference to the types of difficulty they are intended to treat. Finally, we look at a number of different variables which help us decide what sort of approach to take.

The aim of therapy

The aim of therapy will vary according to what the therapist is trying to achieve. Parents often want their child to be 'cured', meaning that they want their child to be *normal*, although it is sometimes unclear exactly what they mean by this. However, it is wrong to assume that you can cure speech and language problems in the same way that you can take away a headache by taking paracetamol. There is often no simple solution and the process requires a great deal of collaboration between therapist, teacher, parent and all the others who have contact with the child. Nevertheless, for some children, it may be practical to think of simply setting them back on the right track. This is particularly true of children up to the age of three or four, many of whom may need minimal assistance to catch up with their peers in nursery. By way of example, Kofi was referred to speech and language therapy at the age of two and a half. He spoke very little, was very distractible and, when tested, had limited verbal comprehension. The therapist concentrated on developing his attention and listening skills. These improved relatively quickly and as a consequence his understanding increased and he was soon speaking as well as other children in the nursery.

However, for others there may be a need to be more realistic and assume that we have to *find* them ways of coping with their difficulties without necessarily assuming that we will remove them altogether. In other words, we teach them to work more effectively with the skills that they have got in order to promote development of those that they do not. This may be done by assessing the child and working on apparent gaps in their knowledge. Thus the therapist might work on vocabulary or specific syntactic structures. Alternatively this may be done by working on their strengths and encouraging them to compensate for other areas of weakness. Thus when children are described as having 'word finding difficulties' it may be more appropriate to think of using their strengths to help themselves to retrieve a word. Hence one child may be helped to think of the sound at the start of the word while another may be helped by being encouraged to think of words which are related in meaning to the one that they are after.

For a small number of children, spoken language may not be a realistic goal in the short term. In such cases it may be appropriate to encourage the child to use other types of communication, what we know as *augmentative communication systems*. These are intended to supplement what the child already uses and allow him to start communicating and thereby reduce his frustration. The intention in many cases is that such systems are introduced at a relatively early stage in the child's education and that they are then withdrawn or become redundant as the child's conventional communication skills develop. Such systems are of three types – manual, technological or simple picture displays.

In many cases the aims of any intervention will not be confined to changing the child's communication skills. If we take the view that language is dependant upon other non-linguistic skills, it is reasonable to argue that promoting those other skills related to language will have a knock-on effect on language development itself. For example, many people argue that one of the areas with which a great many of these children find difficulty is listening and attention, and this must be the focus of therapy on the grounds that children will not be taking in the language that they hear around them until they are able to focus upon it. Similarly, as we have noted in Chapter 2, many authors have highlighted the role of the child's need for symbolic skills underlying language development. One of the most prominent symbolic skills associated with language is play. Many therapists advocate using play as a means of promoting language development. With older children it is similarly important to promote social confidence by providing realistic contexts – e.g. going to the shops and asking for change. In Chapter 9 the Director of AFASIC describes their activity weeks which are designed to promote communication skills by developing the children's confidence.

For many the main area of concern surrounds the child's ability to hold a conversation with others. This may be less of a problem for the younger child who perhaps relates more directly to adults, but as children start to learn in groups, how they relate to one another is likely to be at the heart of their problem. For such children it is often necessary to teach them how to initiate conversations, how to monitor the responses of others and how to repair conversations which have gone wrong. This is important because it is as necessary for their interaction with their peers in class as it is for their contacts with the adults around them. For such children the focus of therapy is likely to be the child's intention to communicate and the prevention of their withdrawal from unsuccessful communications altogether.

Equally, it may be important to take the focus away from the child entirely. In a straightforward way it is obvious that the child is the one with the delay and should be the recipient of any help offered. However, it is also true to say that it is our *response* to that child which may be as important as work with the child himself. Some parents find this difficult to understand but from the point of view of the therapist, we know that the parent of the young child is the person who spends more time than anyone else with the child and may well be the most important person to work with. For example, it may be easier to work with the child at home but via the parent than in the clinic or in a school. This is much more common when we are speaking of younger children than it is when we consider older children. In such cases the therapist's objectives could be to facilitate the communication between parent and child. As we have seen in earlier chapters, language-impaired children can often be very frustrating for parents and they may well benefit from this type of help.

Specific goals – where, when and with whom?

Where?

For many years, work based in clinics or health centres has characterised speech and language therapy with children and especially pre-school children. This has distinct advantages when the child is first seen because it offers the therapist the ideal opportunity to elicit the case history information described in Chapter 3. Such discussion often requires considerable thought on the part of the parent and therapist. Indeed it would be appropriate to describe it as thinking together about the child and his environment. Noisy, busy environments such as schools and nurseries may not be the ideal place for such discussion. It is important that such early sessions should be seen as an ideal opportunity for the parent to air their concerns as much as it is for the therapist to gather information.

Similarly, the clinic can offer the therapist an ideal opportunity to interact with the child without undue distraction from other children. It might be argued that children are best seen interacting with their peers. However, there is much that can be learned from offering a child a range of different toys/materials and monitoring their response in a calm environment. Having parent and child present together can also be helpful. Therapists can observe them together and look for ways to help them to communicate more effectively should the need arise.

From their base in a clinic, many speech and language therapists work in a variety of other settings such as social services day nurseries, schools or child development centres. The setting will play a large part in determining who will be seen and how the therapist will work with each child. Where possible, work with very young children is carried out through the parent. Where this is impractical, extensive use is made of carers or key workers. Many speech and language therapists spend a considerable part of their time working with day-care staff, making suggestions as to how best to help promote speech and language development. In some cases they actually assess and treat children themselves, in others they act as a consultant for those with direct contact with the children.

When the child starts school it may be more practical for the therapist to work directly with the teacher. This is not to deny the importance of the contact with the parent. On the contrary, this remains of primary significance. However, it makes sense to have as many people as possible pulling in the same direction to help a child's communication skills. Given that children spend such a lot of their time in school, this is where there are most opportunities. Influencing the school environment for the child may be more relevant than only focusing on the difficulties within the child. Getting the child's teacher involved can then become a primary goal. Some children in mainstream school will have statements of special educational need as described in Chapters 7 and 10. If this is the case, it is likely that a specific staff member will be allocated to the child in question for a designated number of hours a week. This being the case, the therapist would work with the staff member in question and objectives would be discussed accordingly.

It is likely that therapists working within the framework of the National Curriculum in a mainstream school would use different materials and be working to a different timetable from a therapist working exclusively in a clinic. The objectives for most of this work will be to provide the child with strategies for taking best advantage of the educational system.

Case 1

In one example a five-year-old boy had been treated in clinic for some time. When he started in school the therapist spoke to both his teacher and the classroom assistant to establish carry over between what had been going on in the clinic and the classroom. Like many language-impaired children he experienced considerable difficulties in putting his ideas into a correct sequence. In clinic much of the work had been carried out using educational materials such as picture cards or sequencing activities carried out with toys. In school it was possible to extend the activities to include a number of different aspects of the classroom routine. Thus the classroom assistant specifically focused on the child's sequencing when it came to his number work, when they were recounting the activities of the previous weekend and when the class was asked to follow a given sequence before they went out to play.

When?

A common question raised by parents is that of when you should start offering extra help to children whose language appears to be progressing more slowly than that of other children. In part, this question depends on when you are able to make such decisions and in part it depends on the services that are available.

When is it possible to say that a child is developing at a different speed from other children? Children who are *generally* developmentally delayed are easiest to identify early on because their problems are most apparent. For example, they may also be slow to walk, become toilet trained etc. However, as we have discussed in previous chapters, many children have more specific speech and language difficulties and do not present with such obvious developmental problems. It is much more difficult to pick this group out when they are very young.

Parents sometimes express concern when their child is 18 months old, but when you ask them on what basis they are making that judgement you find that they are making a direct comparison with the child's older brother when he was the same age. It is difficult to make much of this simply because the range of normal language development is so great in the first few years of life. It is true that the two children in question may be very different but it may be that the language skills of the slower child are still within normal limits. Just because one child is behind another does not necessarily mean that they have a problem or need speech and language therapy.

Nevertheless, if we ask parents of children in a language unit, and therefore with pronounced language learning difficulties, when they were first concerned, for many the answer seems to be shortly after the second birthday. This is reflected in what parents said in Chapter 1. Many health authorities do now provide a speech and language therapy service for such young children and it seems likely that this will increase. It is often very difficult to pick out specific types of language difficulty at this age and intervention tends to be of a general nature before the age of two years. However, as the child gets older, the difficulties that he experiences become more clearly defined and the intervention also becomes more focused.

Case 2

Vivek was two when he was first referred for speech and language therapy. His parents were concerned that he was not saying as much as other children. Assessment indicated that although his physical skills were appropriate for his age he had both comprehension and expressive language skills more akin to those of a child of 12 months. Intervention involved providing the parents with strategies for gaining and holding his attention and for ensuring that what they said coincided with what he was looking at at any one time. Despite suggestions, he responded slowly to this help.

Case 3

Mary was four and a half when referred by her parents because she was not talking as much as other children. Assessment indicated that her developmental skills and her receptive language skills were well within the normal range but that she had specific difficulties with the production of sounds and this was affecting how much she could say at any one time. In this case intervention focused on developing her sound system with a view to increasing her syntactic development. Her sound system developed rapidly in therapy and the target of intervention shifted to her expressive language within four months.

The important point to bear in mind here is that both the play materials and the nature of the goals change as the child moves on to nursery and school. There is nothing static about language development and the therapy must reflect this.

With whom?

When we consider who is responsible for providing help for language-impaired children, it is tempting to assume that this will be the speech and language therapist. In fact, much will depend on the circumstances experienced by each child. We can say emphatically that parents will play a major role in helping their children cope with their language difficulties. The same can be said of all the other adults with whom the children come in to contact. The health visitor or clinical medical officer who first sees them may be in a position to give advice at a strategic point. Similarly, nursery teachers and nursery workers will all be providing relevant verbal input to the child and are also likely to be in a good position to respond to the suggestions made by the speech and language therapist. Those working in specific units are likely to be very well informed about the needs of the children in their care. Of course, the child's classroom teacher will have particular responsibility for promoting language development. Again, this is likely to be in conjunction with the speech and language therapist but in practice this is not always the case.

Finally, it is important to bear in mind the role of the assistant. In some cases these will be speech and language therapy assistants. In others they will be general classroom assistants or special needs assistants. Such staff are found throughout the education system and increasingly in the National Health Service. They play a considerable role in helping children develop. Sometimes parents say that they only want their child to be seen by the speech and language therapist because otherwise they will not receive the best attention. Such concerns are generally unwarranted. All assistants work directly under the guidance of either a teacher or a therapist and the work that they are carrying out with your child will have been discussed extensively beforehand. The important point is that the assistants do receive training and support from speech and language therapists together with teachers specialising in this area. If you, as a parent, are in doubt, always ask.

The speech and language therapist should be seen as the facilitator of the process of language development, working alongside others to bring the best out in the child. In some cases contact will be direct, in others indirect. The important point is that, if we interpret the term in its broadest sense, 'intervention' refers to whatever we carry out with the child. The better we can develop strategies that work, the better it will be for the child.

With what?

In recent years a number of shops and outlets have been set up specifically advertising educational materials. These are often very beautifully made and very resilient to the hardest wear that children can inflict on them.

This seems to have led to some parents assuming that such materials are required if a child is to develop properly. While they obviously do provide the children with wonderful opportunities, it is important to stress that when it comes to therapy or intervention it is not the materials so much as what you do with them that counts. Carefully thought out use of simple materials is often more useful than simply buying large quantities of 'educational' materials which are then not used appropriately.

Parents sometimes become worried that toys used in therapy sessions are inappropriate because they are not the same as the ones the child is exposed to at home. For example, they may express concern that the therapist is using dolls with their little boy when they do not feel that it is suitable for little boys to play with dolls. The important factor here is not to become too fixed on the toy itself but to look at what it is being used for. So in this example we need to note that the doll is being used to foster the child's underlying symbolic skills. We are not simply teaching the child to like a given doll. We must always bear in mind what we are using the toy for.

Working with children on their own or in groups

Therapists frequently have to make the decision whether it is better to work with the child on his own or with other children. There are pros and cons with both approaches. Parents often prefer the individual contact, at least in the early stages of intervention, because they feel that their child is getting the attention they need. If their child is seen in a group with many other children, obviously they will not get as much individual attention as they would if they were seen on their own. Of course, individual attention is also important to allow the parent to have plenty of opportunity to raise any questions that they need to address. It depends on the child's age. Very young children – below the age of two years or there abouts – may not cope very well in groups anyway. Thereafter it depends how much the child needs to communicate with other children as to whether a group is most appropriate. In some cases very specific linguistic behaviours may be easier to target in individual sessions. In other cases the child may react badly to other children and a group would increase the child's distress unnecessarily.

However, in many cases groups are seen to be a more natural way for young children to interact, although it is probably a mistake to assume that groups reflect better children's experiences more than individual contact does. This depends clearly on whether the children have brothers or sisters or are in nursery and this needs to be taken into consideration. Groups can make them feel less pressured than they would be if they were surrounded by adults and this may help them to communicate more naturally. Groups can also provide an element of competition between the children which may make them try just that little bit harder. Of course, we have to be careful in assuming that such competition is necessarily a good thing. Many children find this difficult to cope with and we have to be careful in assuming that they will necessarily get on well in a group, as the example below illustrates well.

Case 4

Kevin was three when he was referred for speech and language therapy. He had a history of slow language development but there were no problems apparent from his medical history. He was only using two or three words and seemed very reluctant to speak. He was placed in a group for children of his age with equivalent difficulties. All the children in the group were unsettled when they started often because they had had limited experience of this sort of structure. However, most of the children worked out the rules and the order in which activities took place within three sessions. Kevin not only found predicting what was about to happen difficult but he also reacted badly to the other children. Rather than sitting and watching the others before participating, he deliberately avoided them and showed distress when he was encouraged to join in. In effect, it was not appropriate for him to be in a group because he was not ready to benefit from it. He was consequently taken out of the group and seen on his own and then with one other child.

As children move through the pre-school period in to school, the issues regarding group work change somewhat. Increasingly, children do most of their learning in groups and it becomes more difficult to justify taking them out of their natural groups for special help. They need to learn skills that they can apply in their class and with their friends. We cannot assume that teaching them language skills separately will necessarily carry over into other aspects of their work. And if intervention does not generalise in this way we have to consider its value very seriously.

Therapy approaches

Although intervention is geared towards the needs of the individual child, a number of specific programmes or approaches have been developed. Therapists often refer to these and parents need to be aware of what is available. For example, these approaches, or words taken from them, are sometimes referred to in discussions or in reports, but the terms remain uninformative unless the parent knows to what they refer. Accordingly we touch on a variety of programmes which are currently in use in the UK. The approaches are discussed in greater detail in Law (1994)[1] and the reader is encouraged to go to this text if they would like more information about an approach which is being used for their child.

The Derbyshire Language Scheme (DLS)

The DLS was designed originally for use in schools for children with moderate learning difficulties but has since been very widely applied throughout centres specialising in work with language-delayed children. Children are assessed initially using a short *Rapid Screening Test* and then assessed in more depth using a *Detailed Test of Comprehension*. The testing focuses on the range of meanings that the child is able to comprehend and express. Testing materials include pictures and symbolic play materials (dolls, chairs etc.) and the child is required to carry out the activity under instruction. At each step activities can be modelled and taught at the appropriate level for the child. There are two volumes of activities available as a part of the scheme targeted at areas of difficulty both in expression and comprehension.

The scheme makes extensive use of the *information carrying word (ICW)* (see Chapter 3), a term developed to distinguish between the total number of words in an utterance and the number of words the child needs to know to extract the correct meaning. This depends on the utterance in question and it depends on the syntax. Thus 'put the doll on the chair' has six words in it but this drops to one ICW if there is a choice between a doll and a teddy bear and two if there is also a choice between a chair and a

---

1   See list of useful books p.151–158.

table. Although the scheme starts by emphasising comprehension it progresses to promote expression and makes extensive use of 'role reversals' or situations in which the child is encouraged to make structured verbal demands of adults or other children and take control of the activities themselves. Although the Derbyshire Language Scheme is highly structured it is intended that children use it to learn to communicate naturally.

Living Language

Living Language also includes a screening procedure, in this instance an observation checklist in the pre-verbal booklet covering four categories of development and a vocabulary checklist, filled in by parents or carers, teachers and therapists. The scheme is a language syllabus designed primarily for use in special schools. It offers a guide to the teaching of vocabulary and features of grammar which can be addressed in any and all subject areas. Thus vocabulary development is fostered through the teaching of curriculum topics. Each topic includes a core of nouns and verbs set as teaching objectives. As the children learn to use these, adjectives, adverbs and prepositions are gradually introduced. Vocabulary topics are organised in levels of increasing difficulty reflecting normal language learning between approximately two and seven years. The purpose of the Living Language programme is to promote children's language development through the routines of everyday life and through the children's active involvement with others.

Whereas the Derbyshire Language Scheme is intended for use by speech and language therapists and teachers with special training, Living Language is designed to be used by teachers with the minimal amount of training. Vocabulary is taught systematically and integrated into classroom tasks. The assumption is that with vocabulary comes the desire to communicate more effectively and this generates the more complex language structures.

The Nuffield Dyspraxia Programme

The Nuffield Dyspraxia Programme is intended for use with children who have difficulty coordinating their production of speech sounds can be delivered by speech and language therapists and other staff under their supervision. Thus they may be able to say the sounds on their own, but as soon as they are asked to put them together into words, the sounds get mixed up. Thus the children may be able to say 'p','k','t' in isolation but when they try to say 'potato' it comes out as 'dedado' or 'topapo'. These children are sometimes referred to as 'dyspraxic' (see Chapter 5). This suggests that they have a very serious speech difficulty caused by a difficulty coordinating the speech apparatus. It is worth noting that the value of the term 'dyspraxic' has been questioned by some authors. Nevertheless it continues to be used by many therapists.

The programme starts with a detailed assessment of the speech apparatus (mouth, lips, tongue and palete) both at rest and in movement. Gradually the tasks become more complex and the child is required to move from single sounds to short words and then long words and phrases. Each sound has a corresponding picture and this is used throughout the programme so that the child comes to associate that sound when ever they see the picture in question. Much of the work depends on drilling the child in the production of the required sound sequences.

The Metaphon approach

The Metaphon approach focuses not on the motor aspects of speech but on the child's awareness of the nature of speech sounds. Thus children are encouraged to think about the shape of sounds and about how and where they are produced. For example, are they long like 's' or short like 't', quiet like 'p' or loud like 'b'? Are these made at the front of the mouth such as 'p' or 'b' or at the back of the mouth such as 'k' or 'g'? The emphasis is always, in the first instance, on the perception of the sounds and only when this is well established do the authors suggest that the therapist moves on to the production of the sounds themselves. One interesting dimension which distinguishes this approach from others is that the first phase of the scheme begins by drawing the child's attention to the physical characteristic of sounds through concrete aspects of the child's experience rather than through explicit reference to the sounds themselves. The term 'meta' in the title of the scheme suggests that it is awareness which is the key and that once this is established the children will make the appropriate judgements about the sounds they produce and effectively change their own system. The authors suggest that for most children changes can be noted in a relatively short period of time and in the scheme they provide a set of short tests which can measure change every four weeks or so.

The non-directive approach

For some children the focused work described above is not practical because their attention is too poor or because they become very upset when asked to do things that they find difficult. In such cases it is best to take the emphasis away from speech altogether. If we do not do so we may find that we effectively stop the child from communicating as much as they were already. One approach which has been developed to encourage the child to communicate while placing minimal demands on the child is known as 'non-directive' therapy. In such cases the room is arranged such that there are interesting materials to hand and the child is encouraged to explore that environment for themselves. The therapist effectively takes a back seat in the session and rather than asking questions and directing the child, just comments on what the child is doing 'you are taking out a car, now you are driving it into the garage'. Many children who do not find verbal communication easy appreciate this approach and gradually come to respond to it in a verbal manner. It is sometimes difficult for parents seeing their child involved in such work to understand the objectives. These will need to be clearly identified prior to the start of therapy. Such an approach is usually carried out in environments which are relatively controlled such as the therapy room in a school or a speech and language therapy clinic. Unlike Living Language or the Derbyshire Language Scheme, it is often impractical to carry out this type of work in the more naturalistic setting of a classroom. Therapists who use this technique would argue that such children are not ready to fit into a conventional classroom regime and that the approach helps them to adapt to the spoken voice.

The Hanen Early Language Parent Programme

This approach has been used for many years in Toronto, Canada, but has recently started to make an appearance in the UK. It functions by stressing the role played by the parent and develops strategies for the parents to use at home. Indeed, it is set up so that the therapists work with the parents rather than the children. As mentioned earlier in this chapter, parents may find this rather difficult to understand but the emphasis is placed on the role of the parent in changing the child rather than the same thing being done by a professional. Clearly it is better if parents make their own decisions in this respect. Those designing the Hanen programme have been particularly interested in the way that adults learn and the programme involves all sorts of different ways of teaching parents how to help their children. We cannot assume that all adults pick up new information in the same way and the same is, of course, true of children.

The programme aims to promote a way of interacting with the young child which mirrors normal development. Parents are encouraged to tune in to their child's needs and to avoid imposing their own agenda on the child. We all know how easy it is not to concentrate on the child's needs when we are rushing around. The parent is encouraged to adjust what they say to their child's language level. Again it is all too easy to talk, over children's heads and simply assume that they have picked it up. Finally, parents are encouraged to add information to what the child has said, to extend what they have said. Thus if the child says 'key' the parent might respond 'Yes, it's mummy's key' or if they say 'mummy's key' the parent might expand it 'Yes, mummy's key goes in the lock.' The important point to remember is that the advocates of the Hanen programme are only really suggesting that parents do what parents usually do when they are encouraging their child to speak. But when we have children who find the process difficult, parents have to work especially hard to find the right level and not simply assume that the child's age is what is important.

Augmentative communication

Increasingly, therapists are using augmentative communication to encourage speech and language development in young children. By 'augmentative' we mean systems which support verbal communication. In some cases these will be manual signing systems such as *Makaton, Paget Gorman, finger spelling* and *cued articulation*. In others these may include communication boards which have signs on them such as Rebus or technological communication aids such as a Touch Talker. There is not space to go into the details of these individual systems here, except to say that each system is designed for a specific purpose. In most cases these systems are designed to help the child make sense of communication and then move on to function independently of the augmentative system. The systems are not designed to replace speech and are very unlikely to do so despite some of the apprehensions expressed by parents.

Although these approaches may appear self-contained, children are not simply slotted into one system. There is no one recipe which works for all children. Discussion between parents and therapist leads to an understanding of the child's and the parents' needs and priorities. In the final analysis it should be the skills of the child which determine how we go about our therapy, and for this reason most therapists adopt a mixed approach, for example taking elements of the Derbyshire Language Scheme, but supplementing them with elements from the Living Language Scheme. Of course there are a great many specific techniques which are not a part of any programme at all. They have been developed by individuals through their experience of children with difficulties acquiring language. We must always remember that the motivation of the child is all important and this has to be the place from which all therapy stems.

Factors considered when providing intervention

We saw in Chapter 3 that our decisions about children depend on a variety of factors which we investigate when we first meet with parents. These same factors influence the choices we make when deciding how to help the children.

The age of the child

As indicated in Chapter 2, we know that many of these children start with a general delay in their language development and that their strengths and weaknesses become clearer as they get older. This means that the focus of our intervention will also change as the child ages. Initially we will probably be working on encouraging parents to listen closely to what the child is saying, watch what he is doing and follow the child's lead. We will stress the need to use relevant vocabulary and to make sure that the child is listening to what is being said before we assume that he is able to take it in and make use of it. Later we may ignore certain areas of communication development and home in on others. We may work on specific speech sounds, whole groups of sounds or aspects of grammatical development. For many children the most important issue is whether they can communicate effectively with their peers in school and their friends at home. For this reason the emphasis for many shifts from the grammatical to the social as the child goes up through the school. Whereas it may be of particular importance to teach children in the pre-school period about the way in which verbs function, later on we are more likely to focus on practical skills such as how we ask for something in a shop or how we insist on something without having a tantrum. In school, of course, the activities must fit into the targets set for the National Curriculum.

The type of difficulty experienced by the child

Tests of understanding, expression and speech will tell us where the best place may be to start our intervention. We may eliminate one area and focus on another. The targets of the intervention need to be clear so that we know whether we are trying to bring the child on in one particular area such as phonology or whether we are attempting to use the child's existing strengths to help him compensate for other areas of difficulty. Parents need to make sure that they are familiar with these targets and are able to ascertain whether the child has improved.

As indicated above, it may not be simply a question of taking the child out of the class and working on skills divorced from the classroom activities. It is probably more likely now that speech and language therapists will work in close conjunction with those responsible for classroom activities and blend those activities into the therapy, varying the emphasis according to the needs of the child. For example, if a child with a language difficulty was in a class which was focusing for the term on life cycles in general and those associated with pond life in particular, we might consider using the topic words from the class in the therapy session. If the child had difficulties in understanding tense and sequences of action we could make use of the frog's life cycle to make the therapist's work meaningful. If he or she had difficulties classifying related concepts the speech and language therapist might work on the relationship between mammals, amphibians and insects, looking to see if the child was aware of strategies you could use to sort them into categories. The important point is that different difficulties will demand different solutions. There is little or no reason why those solutions need be kept separate from the classroom activity.

Other associated factors

Although we often attempt to separate speech and language development from the child's other skills so that we can try to assess them, this is often not very realistic. Language is, after all, at the root of most of what we do and nowhere is this more relevant than in the school years. Later on we may choose activities that are more or less verbally demanding but during the school years almost everything we do is affected by those skills. As a result it is virtually impossible to separate language skills from those associated with reading and writing. We know that many children who start with delayed language development are also at risk of finding literacy skills difficult to acquire. Similarly, it is difficult to discuss language skills without also taking into consideration a child's social development. Many children who have difficulties in communicating find interaction with other children hard and they may withdraw from social contact. As a result they may effectively have less experience of how to deal with other children.

Summary

There are a great many options open to speech and language therapists and teachers working with language-impaired children when it comes to promoting a child's language development. In making the choice it is necessary to be clear about what we are trying to achieve and keep a close eye on whether the child is progressing as we would expect. Parents need to play an active role in this process. It is significant that the majority of approaches described above have not been proved to work in the same way that we can show that a particular drug is effective. Therapists and teachers adopt particular techniques and modify how they work as the circumstances and the needs of the child demand.

CHAPTER 9

What Can We Do About It?
The Role of the Independent Sector

The two principal charities in the UK which provide support and resources are Invalid Children's Aid Nationwide (ICAN) and the Association For All Speech Impaired Children (AFASIC). We felt that it would be useful to include some details about these organisations and, rather than write about them ourselves, we have asked representatives from each organisation to do it for us. Brian Jones and Fraser Mackay from ICAN and Norma Corkish from AFASIC describe their respective organisations below.

Invalid Children's Aid Nationwide (ICAN)
Brian Jones and Fraser Mackay

The history

ICAN was established in 1888 (as the Invalid Children's Aid Association) with the motto 'To give everyone a chance'. For over 100 years that motto has held good and we have constantly been involved at the sharp end of service provision for children. Recently the name and the initials have changed and we are now known as Invalid Children's Aid Nationwide (ICAN).

For over 30 years ICAN has been increasingly involved in helping children with speech and language difficulties. In 1958 ICAN opened the John Horniman School in Worthing, Sussex, which focuses on providing for the needs of children between five and ten years of age who are experiencing difficulties acquiring speech and language. Since then teachers and therapists from the school have developed a range of teaching materials which have become widely used as other professionals are increasingly aware of the needs of these children. More recently we have opened Meath School in Ottershaw, Surrey, for children aged between 5 and 12 years and Dawn House School, Rainworth in Nottinghamshire, which concentrates on children from 5 through to 16 years.

Our aims

We can best illustrate what we achieve through the experience of a child recorded by her mother.

> Lucy, aged six years, had a vocabulary of less than 50 words, despite a weekly speech therapy session since the age of four. She had been in mainstream infant school for 18 months with a special needs assistant working with her each morning. In the afternoon she would skip off classes. Staff knew she wasn't being naughty but they were unable to communicate at her level.
>
> The day Lucy was interviewed at Meath was like sun entering a dark room. She met the reception class, where children talked with their hands as well as their voices. Instinctively she recognised her peer group. For us, as her parents, it was a revelation. The day Lucy was given a placement at Meath changed our lives. The intensive speech therapy, backed up by teaching with understanding and a high level of pastoral care, ensured that she progressed socially and emotionally.
>
> The six years at the school worked wonders and she has gone on to board at a secondary school. We look back to when Lucy entered Meath and we look forward hopefully.

Lucy's story is one that has been repeated time and again.

Each of our schools is slightly different in the way in which they work and in the range of children who benefit from a place in them. What they all have in common is well expressed by Jonathan's mother.

> This was the place for our son. Once inside the door, I became aware that, for the first time, here was sympathy and most importantly, complete understanding of the situation and the need for urgency. Here was the place where language and communication skills, school work, and social and emotional development all went hand in hand.

The schools all offer programmes carefully planned by highly trained teachers, speech and language therapists and child-care workers to ensure an intensive and fully integrated language environment.

The headteacher at John Horniman School says:

> We work in partnership with parents to understand each child's difficulties. By providing the highest level of expertise, knowledge and educational programmes, we support the child by nurturing self-esteem and building skills and confidence. As a team we aim to enable each child to become a happy and active member of the school and to enjoy responsibility and interact positively with their peer group at home and within their local communities.

For boarders, support continues as residential child-care staff focus on practical life skills. The schools make full use of facilities within their local communities. Children are also involved in Brownies, Cubs, swimming, trampolining and the like. For day pupils, the schools maintain links with home through a variety of contact mechanisms to ensure that full support is available.

A range of different professionals are involved in each of the schools. These will include occupational therapists and family support workers, educational psychologists and paediatricians, all of whom will be working along side the teaching and speech and language therapy staff. Regular parental visits to the schools are encouraged and the family support workers ensure continuous liaison and mutual support between school and family.

Educationally, children have access to all areas of the National Curriculum at an appropriate level, using cross-curricular topic work and subject-specific teaching. Where appropriate, staff work with the child using the Paget Gorman Signed Speech (PGSS). This recognises that a child has good visual skills and requires a visual means of communication. As the child learns to comprehend through the auditory channel, the need for PGSS slips away and is replaced naturally by speech.

Commenting on PGSS Jonathan's mother says:

> Paget Gorman was to open him up to the pleasure of communication... and with that his spoken language and communication increased daily.

She concludes her description:

How he can talk now! Our phone calls...are now long and detailed... There is rarely a word we cannot understand nor any misunderstanding on his part.

Another parent said of his son:

Once he wouldn't speak. Now, not only can he argue but he often wins!

New directions

There is a move away from residential education today, and this is shown by the high percentage of pupils attending ICAN schools but who do not board. There is also a trend away from providing separate provision for children with speech and language difficulties towards provision in language units in mainstream schools or even total integration into such schools. Sometimes support is available for children in these circumstances. Sometimes it is not.

These two trends have been recognised by ICAN for some time and, indeed, they have much about them which we support. However, we believe that the nature of the provision combined with the level of need means that specific schools will continue to be necessary in some cases. Further, we believe that considerable input into many of the language units around the country is needed to maximise benefit to the children involved. We are doing this through providing training for professionals and some consultancy to local authorities.

We are also beginning to work with Local Education Authorities in secondary schools, offering support to small groups of teenagers who have specific speech and language difficulties. The expertise we have developed in this field is exemplary and this is an important way for us to offer help to the widest possible number of children.

We have also recognised the considerable part to be played by nursery education in the provision for speech- and language-impaired children. We have opened a number of such nurseries which work specifically with children with speech and language difficulties while integrating them into the work of the mainstream nursery. In these nurseries we are concentrating on providing intensive speech and language therapy which focuses on the child's development of receptive and expressive language, vocabulary, attention and the ways in which a sound is formed. Parents are also advised on how to reinforce these skills at home. Children work in small groups in a stimulating and relaxed environment and also benefit from interaction with children in the rest of the nursery.

Information, advice and support

ICAN also has an information department based at its head office, which can provide a range of answers to queries from parents and professionals alike. Through the information department we can also offer a range of publications which have been developed by us and which are available to therapists and teachers to support them in their work. We can also provide a list of all the language units in the UK. Through our specialist training centre, we are now offering a range of training for speech and language therapists, teachers and classroom assistants from mainstream schools and language units. Course details are again available from our head office. In addition, questions specifically related to the ICAN schools can be addressed to any of the schools or to ICAN head office.

'I CAN' is one of the most positive phrases we can use. We like to think that it sums up both our approach to our work and, we hope, the children to theirs.

The Association for All Speech Impaired Children
Norma Corkish

The history

AFASIC was founded in 1968 by a speech and language therapist, Margaret Greene. In her work as a therapist she became increasingly concerned about the ignorance of speech and language impairments among doctors, psychologists and education officers and therefore the lack of help available, particularly in the pre-school years, for such children. She decided that an association was needed to improve awareness and one that was run by parents in order that cases could be made most strongly. Soon after the inauguration of the association a parent, Elizabeth Browning, published a book about her struggles in bringing up a son with a specific speech and language impairment entitled *I can't see what you're saying*. Her story told movingly of the difficulties her family faced in obtaining an accurate diagnosis and appropriate educational help and illustrated clearly the importance of the role of parents in securing their child's future. Elizabeth Browning agreed to join the association's Execu-tive Committee and soon became its Chair. She remained Chair for 18 years and under her guidance the association developed into a well-established parent-led body supporting parents and making cases to central and local government on behalf of those children said to have a specific language impairment – i.e. not the result of physical or intellectual disabilities.

AFASIC is a membership organisation, with approximately 1600 members, the majority of whom are parents. A number of these parents are responsible for running AFASIC local groups, of which there are about 50 throughout the United Kingdom. All of the groups provide parents with mutual support but they perform different roles according to the needs of those involved. Some fundraise and organise conferences, workshops and leisure activities for the children and young people. Others liaise with their local authorities for improvements in local provision, such as nursery classes and language units. The level of activity within the groups varies considerably, but each is free to decide its own priorities and choose its own activities within the association's overall brief. The groups are organised into 15 regions. Each region is able to nominate a representative to sit on the Management Committee, which is responsible for developing and monitoring AFASIC's objectives. AFASIC is, therefore, very much a parent-led organisation. At the same time we liaise closely with professionals at both local and national level and many contribute significantly to AFASIC's work.

Over the last five years the association has widened its brief to represent young people as well as children. In addition, it speaks on behalf of *all* those with a speech and language impairment, whether or not they are the result of physical or intellectual disabilities. However, having said that, those with specific speech and language impairment remain at the heart of its work.

Our aims

These are to provide: information, advice and support for parents and professionals, whether members or not, and to increase awareness and recognition of speech and language impairments in order to ensure improvements in educational provision, training for professionals and employment opportunities for the children.

AFASIC group activities are seen as very important to the strength of the organisation and over the next five years the intention is to extend their work with support from the centre.

Information, advice and support

The central office comprises a small group of paid staff, among whom are one national and one regional development officer, who have specific responsibility for developing the work of local and regional groups. Parents and professionals ring or write with a variety of questions. Some parents are particularly interested in knowing the meaning of terms such as 'dyspraxia', 'phonological difficulties' or 'semantic and pragmatic impairments'. Others are interested in how they can help their child and ensure appropriate professional help, especially speech and language therapy. Some are eager to talk to other parents. Others want to know where they can get a second opinion.

Example 1: responding to an individual

Mrs X rang AFASIC to say that she had been told that her three-year-old son, Peter, had pragmatic difficulties and to ask what this meant. She did not know of any other parent whose child had similar difficulties and felt, therefore, very isolated. What could we do to help? We were able to send her some literature on speech and language impairments in general, and pragmatic difficulties in particular, and to give her the name of her local AFASIC group secretary. Mrs X became a member of AFASIC and immediately began to feel less isolated and to regain her confidence.

She contacted us again when a draft statement had been written and asked if we could advise her on certain aspects that concerned her. She sent it to us and following discussion and correspondence with us was able to make the case successfully for additional teaching support and speech and language therapy for Peter's mainstream placement.

Individual advice is given over the phone and by letter to parents and professionals. We provide additional support to members by taking up their cases, if necessary, with their local authorities, though we are not able to be with them at meetings and appeals.

AFASIC produces a considerable amount of literature, which is available through central office and local groups. This literature covers, for example, definitions of speech and language impairments, how parents and professionals can help from pre-school age through to advice on children leaving school, and information on legislation and the National Curriculum. We are also able to advise parents on where they might gain second opinions and provide information on schools that specialise in speech and language impairments.

We publish a newsletter three times a year for members, which provides an opportunity for parents to tell their stories and includes up-dates on legislation, research, technology, publications and courses. We organise annual conferences, seminars and workshops nationally and locally for parents and professionals. Recent themes have included legislative changes, educational provision, pre-school children and working with families. We also host international symposia for professionals.

In addition, activity weeks are run nationally and locally throughout the UK for AFASIC members. These, mostly residential, weeks are usually organised locally and run by parents via the AFASIC groups. They all rely heavily on volunteer staff, many of whom are speech and language therapy students. They began in 1973 and provide challenges outside school and the family. One of the aims of the weeks is to provide an environment in which the children and young people gain self-confidence and improve their communication skills. This is done by providing a number of challenges, many of which are not dependant upon communication skills, such as canoeing, abseiling and walking, and at which the youngsters can succeed. There is a high adult : child ratio to ensure that each child receives plenty of individual support and encouragement.

The weeks are held during the summer and each caters for about 15 children or young people. A total of 90 youngsters benefit each year and many return year after year. One youngster, with a fear of heights and in his eleventh year, was determined to abseil for the first time. He did and his self-confidence improved immensely as a result. We are beginning to involve the young people in the planning of their own weeks, some of which are abroad, and encourage their participation in those for the younger children.

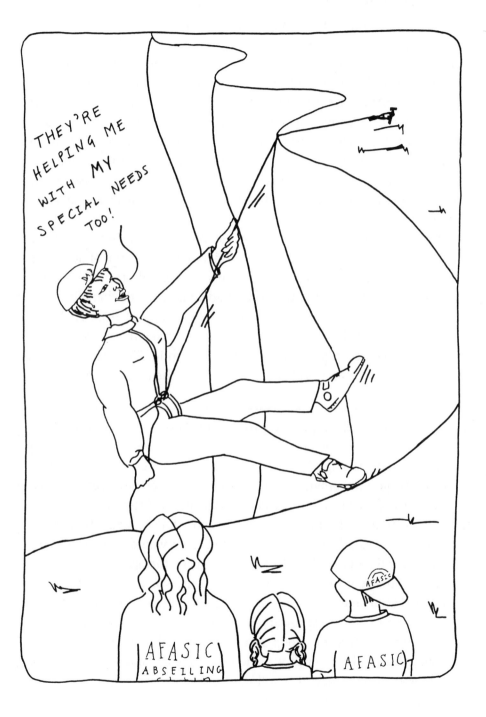

Figure 5

Increasing awareness, and liaison with central and local government

AFASIC is a catalyst for change and an organisation that draws both central and local government's attention to the needs of those with speech and language impairments. It has always been aware of the vital importance of early diagnosis and speech and language therapy. Over the last few years AFASIC has pressed government to ensure improved provision of speech and language therapy within education and has played a key role in ensuring government acknowledgement that speech and language therapy in the majority of cases is educational provision. This work continues and in this our parents play a vital part by making cases to their local authorities, councillors and MPs, both as individuals and as part of our local groups.

AFASIC is very much aware that our parents, both individually and collectively, have vested in them a considerable knowledge of and expertise in speech and language impairments. A key role for AFASIC is to ensure that parents can use this to best advantage for the benefit of their child and the adult that child becomes. With support from AFASIC, a number of parents have had the confidence to make their case and in so doing have secured appropriate help for their child. Similarly we wish to ensure that the young people are able to make their own cases for help.

Example 2: responding to the needs of a local group

Just over ten years ago in one of the Home Counties, where there was no language unit provision, one of the local therapists became very conscious of the need for such a unit and so decided to contact AFASIC. At a meeting of the therapist, parents and AFASIC staff, the parents decided that as a local group of AFASIC they would attempt to raise money for the salary of a speech and language therapist on the understanding that the local educational authority would provide teaching staff and accommodation and that the health authority would, after two years, fund the therapist's salary. Both health and education authorities agreed to this and the group successfully raised a significant sum of money, the result of which was the first language unit in their county. The level of awareness that followed was such that other units were opened in other parts of the county.

The strength gained by the parents in undertaking their fundraising and achieving their target was such that they have continued to support each other and ensured that further units have opened as their children have grown up. In addition, they run local activity weeks, a pre-school group and conferences, and demonstrate quite clearly what a group of parents can achieve.

A number of our groups have been responsible for the opening of the first language unit in their area, for more units as more children are identified, and for follow-on units as the children outgrow the first. In some instances, groups have raised money to help staff or equip such units.

We also continue to stress to central government the importance of appropriate teacher training. AFASIC initiated the first full-time course in the field and have been instrumental in ensuring the development of further courses. We are particularly concerned to ensure that all teachers have an opportunity to learn about speech and language difficulties and the ways to overcome them, both in their initial education and through in-service training.

We see the National Curriculum as providing opportunities for those with communication difficulties with its emphasis on speaking and listening, reading and writing, and point to the fact that almost all children with special educational needs have communication difficulties of one kind or another. Because of this we have worked closely with a number of other organisations, both voluntary and professional, in order to state our cases as strongly as possible.

All of the above helps to increase awareness and recognition, as do the various conferences, seminars and workshops we organise and in which we participate. In addition, publicity is sought, and often gained, in the media – TV, radio, newspapers, magazines and journals, both popular and specialist. At the end of 1993 we were fortunate to have *The Times* write a series of articles about those we represent and our work, along with an appeal for funds.

Future directions

While there have been significant gains in terms of awareness, under-standing and provision since the association was formed in 1968, many challenges remain. This is clear from the continuing stream of calls for help we get from both parents and professionals. Elizabeth Browning's account of over 20 years ago still tells a familiar story for many families today.

In meeting these challenges, the children and young people with speech and language impairments, and the families of which they are a part, will remain the focus of our work. At the same time, in order to meet our objectives most effectively, we hope our local and regional parent-led groups will extend their activities and that we can strengthen our links with other organisations.

CHAPTER 10

The Law and the Language-Impaired Child

Sheila Denney

Parents of children who have special educational needs look for clear information and understanding of their child's needs and guidance as to how best to provide for them. Much of this rests on current legislation and in particular the Education Act (1993). This chapter examines this legislation, discusses what is known as the 'Code of Practice' and goes on to identify procedures which parents can use to obtain what they need for their child should they not agree with what has been allocated. We have also included a copy of the stages of assessment at the back of the book, together with a copy of a statement of special educational need.

Legislation and special educational needs

The 1993 Education Act is largely a replacement of the 1981 Education Act and repeats many of its clauses. It requires the Secretary of State to issue a Code of Practice. This in turn requires education authorities, the governing bodies of all maintained schools and all those who work with children with special educational needs (SEN) including the health and social services to 'have regard' to the code.

The Code of Practice on the identification and assessment of SEN has been approved by parliament and came into effect on 1 September 1994. Those who must have regard to the code must fulfil their duties as prescribed, but some flexibility is maintained in that it is up to them to decide how they wish to do so. It could be unrealistic to expect all authorities or schools to have procedures matching those set out in the Code immediately in place. It is, however, reasonable to expect schools to have planned their position in the light of the Code. Schools have regulations which state that they must publish information on their SEN policies by 1 August 1995 and report to parents on the implementation of these policies in the first annual report published after that date.

In asking 'has the child any special educational needs?', we want to know:

1. Has he a greater difficulty in learning than the majority of children of the same age?

2. Does he have a disability which prevents or hinders him from making use of the educational facilities provided in a local mainstream school for children of the same age within the same area of the educational authority in which he lives?

3. Whether the child is under five years and falls within the definition of 1. or 2. or would do so if special educational provision was not made.

Schools are usually able to meet the needs of the vast majority of children, some with support from external services but not requiring a statutory assessment. About two per cent of children will have special educational needs requiring different or additional provision to that normally made available in a mainstream school. The education authority may then arrange a statutory assessment and special educational provision for a child by means of a statutory statement of special educational needs.

The knowledge, views and experience of parents are vital and effective. Appropriate assessment and provision will come about when there is partnership between parents and their children, their schools, education authorities and other agencies such as health and social services. The Code of Practice will ensure that all maintained schools must draw up a special needs policy, publish it and keep the special educational provision under review. The school's policy will provide parents with a useful check list and a general guide when considering a school for their child. The Code of Practice is a guide for schools and when describing a child's educational difficulties the focus should be on the individual's special educational needs rather than 'categories of handicap'. This is because the children with the same diagnostic label may indeed share a 'condition' but may require very different educational provision. Labels or categories can be useful in grouping children together whose needs arise from a common problem, and are, therefore, likely to have similar needs, though they may be of a very different degree.

Each school will have a named special educational needs coordinator (SENCO) responsible for the day-to-day operation of their special educational needs policy. They will be able to provide information to parents about the school's policy for identification, assessment and provision for all pupils with SEN. The SENCO will also be able to discuss with parents how children with SEN can be integrated within the school as a whole and describe the allocation of resources to and among pupils with SEN and detail their arrangements for the child's educational needs to be met in partnership with parents.

The governing body of the school has a duty to understand issues concerning SEN and must report on the success of the school's SEN policy and how resources have been allocated to and among children with special educational needs over the year.

Identification and assessment

The importance of early identification, assessment and provision for any child who may have special educational needs cannot be over-emphasised. The earlier action is taken, the more responsive the child is likely to be and the more readily can intervention be started. If a child's difficulties prove less responsive to provision made by the school, then an early start can be made in considering the additional or different provision that may be needed to support the child's progress.

In identifying children with special educational needs the school will consider assessment of children within the National Curriculum, especially the pupil's achievements and progress. To provide help to children who have special educational needs, schools should adopt a staged response.

The Code sets out a five-stage model and responsibility for assessing children's needs, Stages 1–3, lies within the school. The educational authority and outside agencies will be closely involved at Stage 3 and the school and the authority share responsibility at Stages 4 and 5.

Some schools and LEAs may adopt different models. It is not essential that there should be five stages and it does not mean that all children will pass through all five stages. It may be sufficient for the school to make provision for children at Stage 1, but a number of children may fail to progress with support at this stage and for such children the school should then move on to Stage 2.

If a child's needs require action at Stages 2 or 3, even if no action has been previously taken at Stage 1, then action should be taken. Records should be properly kept at each stage by the school and if a child is referred for a statutory assessment they should make available to the LEA a record of the school's work with the child. The effective implementation of this will be possible only if schools create positive working relationships with parents and their children and other services. Many children with special educational needs have a range of difficulties and there needs to be effective partnership between all concerned.

The Code of Practice places a responsibility on all schools that they should recognise the importance of consulting parents whether or not their child has special educational needs. All schools should have regard that provision for a child with special needs should match the nature of his or her needs.

- There should be careful recording of a child's special educational needs, the action taken and the outcome.

- Consideration should be given to the ascertainable wishes and feelings of the child.

- There should be close consultation and partnership with parents.

- Outside specialists should be involved and schools should work in close partnership with the providers of such services as they can play an important part in the very early identification of special educational needs and in advising schools on effective provision which can prevent the development of more significant needs.

The SEN coordinator working with the child's class teachers or year tutor and any other relevant specialists are responsible for drawing up the individual educational plan. This plan should build on the curriculum the child is following alongside other pupils and should make use of programmes, activities, materials and assessment techniques readily available to the child's teachers. The plan should usually be implemented, at least in part, in the normal classroom setting

Stages of assessment

STAGE 1

Stage 1 identifies a child's special educational needs and consults with parents and child; the SEN coordinator will register the child's special educational needs, collect relevant information about the child, monitor and review the child's progress and may give some additional help. A date for review should be fixed. This might be within the term.

STAGE 2

Stage 2 is characterised by producing an individual educational plan. The SENCO continues to collect information from other sources, such as from the health services, ensures that the parents are kept informed and takes responsibility for coordinating the child's special educational provision, working with the teacher.

STAGE 3

Stage 3 is characterised by the involvement of specialists from outside the school, such as educational psychologists, speech and language therapists and advisory/support teachers. The school continues to ensure an individual educational plan is drawn up and liaises closely with the parents. Should the child not be progressing at this stage, outside specialist help such as the educational psychologist will help the school to consider whether the child is likely to meet the criteria for statutory assessment by the LEA.

STAGE 4

If a child continues to have special educational needs which appear to require different or additional provision from that already made available, the LEA will consider the need for a statutory assessment and, if appropriate, make a multidisciplinary assessment. All involved, professionals and parents will submit information to the LEA about the child in the form of a written report known as *Advice*.

STAGE 5

The LEA considers the need for a statement of special educational needs after considering information obtained through the educational advice submitted. If appropriate, the LEA will make a statement and arrange, monitor and review the special educational provision.

Parents may make use of *a named person* to assist them in making their case to the education authority. Indeed, Part 3 of the Code specifically recommends that LEAs and parents might discuss the identity of the named person at the start of the assessment process. Some parents may decide not to name a person at this early stage and they do not have to name one. An LEA may see it as their duty to suggest a support group or association should parents wish to contact them.

The statement of special educational needs

Part 1: Introduction.

Part 2: This is a description of the child's specific special educational needs. Parents should ensure that this part adequately reflects all the child's needs as this will inevitably prescribe the level and type of provision made within Part 3.

Part 3: This should specify the short- and long-term objectives which the special educational provision made for the child aims to meet. Educational provision should specify all the educational provision which the authority considers appropriate to meet the needs identified in Part 2. In particular it should note:

1. Any appropriate facilities and equipment, staffing arrangements and curriculum.

2. Any appropriate modifications to the application of the National Curriculum.

3. Any appropriate exclusions to the application of the National Curriculum in detail, and the provision to substitute for any exclusions, in order to maintain a broad and balanced curriculum.

4. Where residential school is appropriate.

Part 4: The type of school which the authority considers appropriate and the name of the school for which the parent has expressed a preference and the name of the school which the authority considers would be appropriate for the child.

Part 5: Here will be specified the non-educational needs of the child for which the authority considers provision is necessary if the child is to benefit properly from the special educational provision specified in Part 3.

Part 6: Here will be specified any non-educational provision which the education authority proposes to make available through a health authority, social services or some other body.

All statements must be reviewed annually. An important formal multidisciplinary review will take place at 14 years of age or shortly thereafter. The first annual review after the young person's 14th birthday and any subsequent reviews until the child leaves school should include a transition plan which will draw together information from a range of individuals within and beyond the school. Under Sections 5 and 6 of the Disabled Persons Act 1986, at the first annual review after the child's 14th birthday, LEAs must seek information from social services departments as to whether a child with a statement under Part 3 of the Education Act (1993) is disabled and may require services from the local authority when leaving school. LEAs should also consult child health services, educational psychologists and any therapists who may have a contribution to make. Parents are asked to contribute what they expect of their son's or daughter's adult life and what they can contribute in terms of helping their child. Some children with statements will remain the responsibility of the authority until they are 19.

Special educational needs tribunal

If a parent disagrees with the LEA, who may refuse to make a formal assessment of their child's needs or refuse to issue a statement of their child's special educational needs or make changes to an existing statement, then first parents should try and discuss this at a local level. If you cannot reach an agreement you can appeal to your local tribunal.

There are certain things tribunals cannot do. They cannot deal with a complaint, for instance, if it seems the LEA are taking a long time to carry out an assessment of your child, or the description in the statement of your child's non-educational needs, or how the LEA plan to meet these, or the way your child's needs are being met at school – the way forward in these instances is to discuss your concerns with your child's school or the LEA or both, and you can take a friend or someone who can help you along with you if you wish to do so.

If you remain unhappy after that then you can write 'and complain' to the Secretary of State For Education at the Department of Education, Sanctuary Buildings, Great Smith Street, London SW1P 3BT or if you live in Wales you can write to the Secretary of State for Wales at the Welsh

Office for Education Department, Government Buildings, Ty Glas Road, Llanishan, Cardiff CF4 5WF.

You can appeal to the tribunal:

1. If the LEA refuses to make a 'statutory assessment' of your child's special educational needs or refuses to issue a statement of your child's special educational needs after making a formal assessment.

2. If the LEA has made a statement or changed a previous one. You can appeal against a) the description in the statement of your child's special educational needs, b) the description in the statement of the special educational provision that the LEA thinks your child should get.

3. If the school named in the statement for your child is not the parent's preference or the LEA has not named a school in the statement.

4. You can also appeal if the LEA refuses to change the name of the school named in the statement.

5. If the LEA refuses to re-assess your child's special educational needs if they have not made a new assessment for at least six months.

6. If the LEA decides not to maintain a statement of your child's needs.

For details of the special educational needs tribunal and to obtain a form to appeal, parents can write to: Special Needs Tribunal, 71 Victoria Street, London SW1, 0171 925 6925.

Parents make an appeal on the form supplied and the tribunal office decides whether the tribunal can deal with the appeal. If they cannot, then parents should hear within ten working days. If they can, then the tribunal office forwards the LEA a copy of the appeal within ten working days and the LEA replies within 20 working days, a copy of their reply is sent to the parents. If they want to make their views known in reply they must do so within 15 working days.

At the same time, the tribunal office will send parents and the LEA a form asking for details of whom they want to attend. Parents and LEA return these forms to the tribunal office within the 30 working days.

During this 30 days any documents and reports can be sent by both parties to the tribunal office. Notice of attendance for the hearing is given at least ten working days beforehand.

A tribunal is made up of three people who will hear the case. The chairman is a lawyer. You do not have to attend the hearing, but it is better to do so as the tribunal members would like to hear what you have to say and you can ask questions. You can send someone to attend on your behalf if you are unable to attend. Parents can bring a friend or representative. There is no legal aid for a solicitor or barrister to represent you. Your child can attend the hearing and answer questions as a witness and you can bring two witnesses to the tribunal, but parents must advise the tribunal who they are. A number of tribunals will be held in London and parents will be paid travelling expenses. The hearing will be as informal as possible with all concerned; tribunal members, yourself and the LEA, being allowed to ask questions. After the hearing you may be asked to wait for the chairman to tell you the decision. Otherwise parents will receive an answer within ten days.

Whatever the decision reached, parents and the LEA must accept it. Both the LEA concerned and the parents have the right to appeal in the High Court against the tribunal's decision, not only on points of law. The LEA must keep to the tribunal decision. If they do not do so then parents have the right to complain to the Secretary of State for Education in England and Wales. Addresses of voluntary associations who can help, if you have no friend or representative, are available from both LEA offices and health centres.

The decision not to issue a statement: the note in lieu

Sometimes a statutory assessment process leads an LEA to the conclusion that the child's special educational needs can be met from within the school's own resources, with or without the intervention of professional help from outside the school. In such cases, parents may be very disappointed and see it as a denial of additional resources for their child. When this does occur the LEA can consider issuing what is known as a *note in lieu* of a statement.

In such a note the LEA should set out their reasons for not issuing a statement, and writing a comprehensive and useful note in lieu will require as much thought and time as writing a proposed statement. There may be advantages in the format of the note in lieu which broadly follows the statutory format of the statement, though the different legal status of the two documents must be made absolutely clear. The lay out of a note in lieu is a matter for the educational authority concerned. The first part could describe the child's needs with supporting evidence from the formal assessment. The second part might set out the LEA's reasons for not issuing a statement and offer guidance as to the educational provision which might appropriately be made for the child. The third part might, then again, reflect the advice received and agreement between the LEA and agencies concerned describing any non-educational needs and appropriate provision.

Summary

We have outlined the legal processes involved in legislation and the statutory assessment and statementing of children with SENs. We have also touched upon the tribunal process. It is, of course, to be hoped that parents, education authorities, health and social services and other agencies will work together for the benefit of the child and that, as a parent, you will not need to have recourse to the law. Having said that, the law is, in essence, there to help your child reach his or her potential. As we saw in Chapter 1, parents' experiences do not always match up with what is intended. For this reason it is most important that every parent is well informed.

Useful Books

A great many books have been written about the subject of the difficulties that children experience in acquiring language. Many are very technical and would be unlikely to meet the needs of most parents. Below we include some of the more accessible.

If you do want to do more reading on the subject we would highly recommend your starting by looking at the material produced by AFASIC. They have had a lot of experience in producing materials for parents.

AFASIC (1993) *Alone and anxious.* Available from AFASIC, 347 Central Markets, Smithfield, London EC1.

Browning, E. (1972) *I can't see what you are saying.* East Wittering: Angel Books. Available from AFASIC.

Byers-Brown, B. and Edwards, M. (1989) *Developmental disorders of language.* London: Whurr.

Byrne, R. (1983) *Lets talk about stammering.* London: Allen and Unwin.

Capelin, S. (1993) *Rachel: the 'write' to speak.* Available from Sandra Capelin, Mount Pleasant, Darite, Liskeard, Cornwall PL14 5JW.

Cooke, J. and Williams, D. (1985) *Working with children's language.* Available from Winslow Press, Telford Road, Bicester, Oxon OX6 OTS.

Crystal, D. (1987) *The Cambridge Encyclopaedia of language.* Cambridge: Cambridge University Press.

Harris, J. (1990) *Early language development – implications for clinical and educational practice.* London: Routledge.

Haynes, C. and Naidoo, S. (1991) *Children with specific language impairment.* Oxford: Mackeith Press.

Jeffree, D. and McConkey, R. (1986) *Let me speak.* London: Souvenir Press.

Kersner, M. and Wright, J. (1993) *How to manage communication problems in young children.* Available from Winslow Press, Telford Road, Bicester, Oxon OX6 OTS.

Law, J. (ed) (1994) *Before school: a handbook of approaches to intervention with preschool language impaired children.* Available from AFASIC, 347 Central Markets, Smithfield, London EC1.

Lees, J. (1993) *Children with acquired aphasias.* London: Whurr Publishers.

Manolson, A. (1992) *It takes two to talk – A parent's guide to helping children communicate.* Toronto: Hanen Centre Publications. Available from Winslow Press, Telford Road, Bicester, Oxon OX6 OTS.

Useful Addresses

Here are some addresses which you may find helpful. Many are national centres but you can telephone them for advice and information.

AFASIC
347 Central Markets
Smithfield
London EC1A 9NH
Tel: 0171 236 3632
Fax: 0171 236 8115

British Stammering Association
15 Old Ford Road
London E2 9PJ
Tel: 0181 981 8818
Fax: 0181 983 3591

British Dyslexia Association
98 London Road
Reading
Berkshire RG1 5AU
Tel: (01734) 668271
Fax: (01734) 351927

Child's Play International Ltd
Ashworth Road
Bridgemead, Swindon
Wiltshire SN5 7YD
Tel: (01793) 616286
Fax: (01793) 512795

Contact a Family
170 Tottenham Court Road
London W1P 0HA
Tel: 0171 383 3555
Fax: 0171 383 0259

The Dyspraxia Trust
8 West Alley
Hitchin
Hertfordshire SG5 1EG
Tel: (01462) 454986

Fragile X Society
53 Winchelsea Lane
Hastings
East Sussex TN35 4LG
Tel: (01424) 813147

Invalid Children's Aid Nationwide (ICAN)
Barbican City Gate
1–3 Dufferin Street
London EC1Y 8NA
Tel: 0171 374 4422
Fax: 0171 374 2762

The Independent Panel for Special
Education Advice (IPSEA)
22 Warren Hill Road
Woodbridge
Suffolk IP12 4DU
Tel: (01394) 382814

National Autistic Society
276 Willesden Lane
London NW2 5RB
Tel: 0181 451 1114
Fax: 0181 451 5865

National Children's Bureau
8 Wakley Street
London EC1V 7QE
Tel: 0171 278 9441
Fax: 0171 278 9512

Network 81
1–7 Woodfield Terrace
Stanstead
Essex CM24 8AJ
Tel: (01279) 647415

The Paget Gorman Society
3 Gipsy Lane
Headington
Oxford OX3 7PT
Tel: (01865) 61908

The Royal College of Speech and
Language Therapists
7 Bath Place
Rivington Street
London EC2A 3DR
Tel: 0171 613 3855
Fax: 0171 613 3854

Royal Society for Mentally Handicapped
Children and Adults (Mencap)
123 Golden Lane
London EC1Y 0RT
Tel: 0171 454 0454

SCOPE
The Cerebral Palsy Helpline
PO Box 833
Milton Keynes
Bucks MK14 6DR
Tel: 0800 626216
Fax: (01908) 691702

Stages of Identification and Assessment of Special Educational Needs

Stage 1: class or subject teachers identify or register a child's special educational needs and, consulting the school's SEN coordinator (see Glossary), take initial action.

Stage 2: the school's SEN coordinator takes lead responsibility for gathering information and for coordinating the child's special educational provision, working with the child's teachers.

Stage 3: teachers and the SEN coordinator are supported by specialists from outside the school.

Stage 4: the LEA considers the need for a statutory assessment and, if appropriate, makes a multidisciplinary assessment.

Stage 5: the LEA considers the need for a statement of special educational needs and, if appropriate, makes a statement and arranges, monitors and reviews provision.

School-based Stages: Stage 1

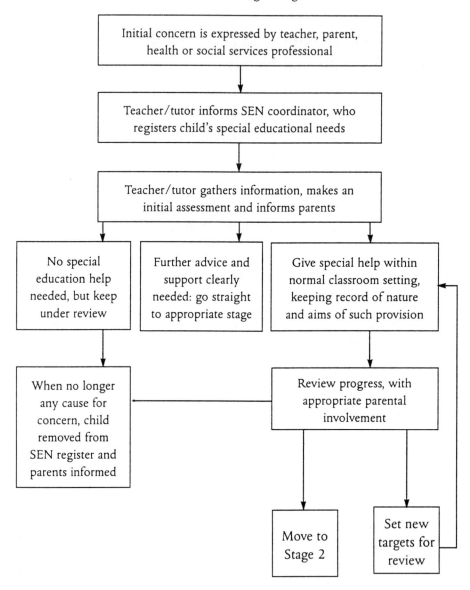

School-based Stages: Stage 2

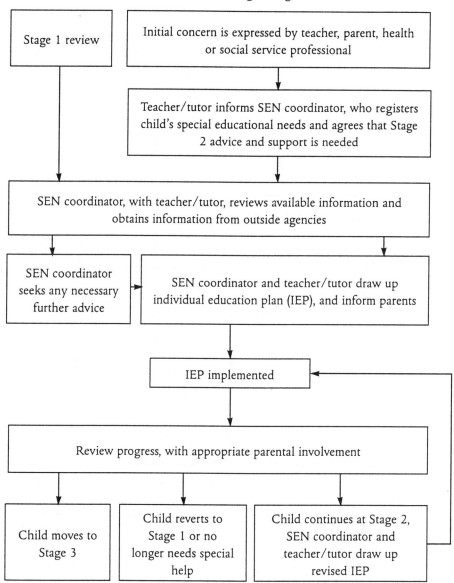

School-based Stages: Stage 3

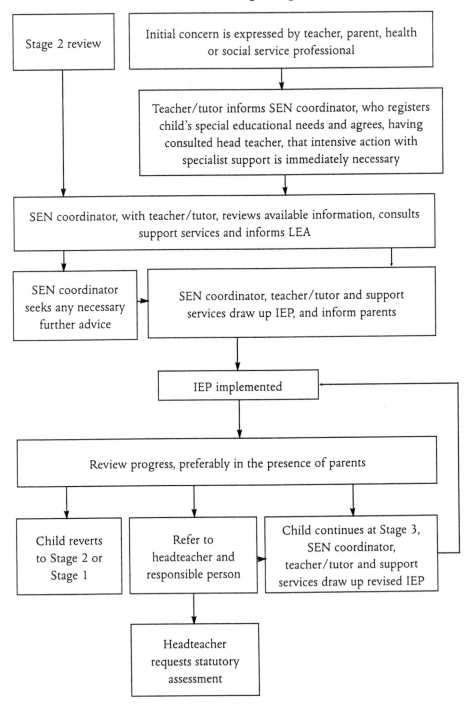

Statement of Special Educational Needs

Part 1: Introduction

1. In accordance with section 168 of the Education Act 1993 ('the Act') and the Education (Special Educational Needs) Regulations 1994 ('the Regulations'), the following statement is made by [*here set out name of authority*] ('the authority') in respect of the child whose name and other particulars are mentioned below.

Child

Surname   Other names

Home address

                                Sex

                                Religion

Date of Birth   Home language

Child's parent or person responsible

Surname   Other names

Home address

                                Relationship to child

Telephone No.

---

2. When assessing the child's special educational needs the authority took into consideration, in accordance with regulation 10 of the Regulations, the representations, evidence and advice set out in the Appendices to this statement.

Part 2: Special educational needs

[*Here set out the child's special educational needs, in terms of the child's learning difficulties which call for special educational provision, as assessed by the authority.*]

Part 3: Special educational provision

Objectives

[*Here specify the objectives which the special educational provision for the child should aim to meet.*]

Educational provision to meet needs and objectives

[*Here specify the special educational provision which the authority consider appropriate to meet the needs specified in Part 2 and to meet the objectives specified in this Part, and in particular specify –*

(a)   *any appropriate facilities and equipment, staffing arrangements and curriculum,*

(b)   *any appropriate modifications to the application of the National Curriculum,*

(c)   *any appropriate exclusions from the application of the National Curriculum, in detail, and the provision which it is proposed to substitute for any such exclusions in order to maintain a balanced and broadly based curriculum; and*

(d)   *where residential accommodation is appropriate, that fact.*]

Monitoring

[*Here specify the arrangements to be made for –*

(a)   *regularly monitoring progress in meeting the objectives specified in this Part,*

(b)   *establishing targets in furtherance of those objectives,*

(c)   *regularly monitoring the targets referred to in (b),*

(d)   *regularly monitoring the appropriateness of any modifications to the application of the National Curriculum, and*

(e)   *regularly monitoring the appropriateness of any provision substituted for exclusions from the application of the National Curriculum.*

Here also specify any special arrangements for reviewing this statement.]

Part 4: Placement

[*Here specify -*

(a)   *the type of school which the authority consider appropriate for the child and the name of the school for which the parent has expressed a preference or, where the authority are required* to specify the name of a school, the name of the school which they consider would be appropriate for the child and should be specified, or

(b) the provision for his education otherwise than at a school which the authority consider appropriate.]

Part 5: Non-educational needs

[*Here specify the non-educational needs of the child for which the authority consider provision is appropriate if the child is to properly benefit from the special educational provision in Part 3.*]

Part 6: Non-educational provision

[*Here specify any non-educational provision which the authority propose to make available or which they are satisfied will be made available by a district health authority, a social services authority or some other body, including the arrangements for its provision. Also specify the objectives of the provision, and the arrangements for monitoring progress in meeting those objectives.*]

_____   _____

Date   A duly authorised officer of the authority

Glossary

The following are some terms used both in this book and by professionals.

Age equivalent
Comes from the use of standardised tests and refers to the average age at which children receive a given score. Thus a five-year-old receives a score equivalent to that of a three-year-old. The concept is widely used by therapists but we have to be careful in interpreting what it means. A five-year-old and a ten-year-old with an age equivalent score of a three-year-old are unlikely to use language in the same way.

Anoxia
A lack of sufficient oxygen to the brain.

Articulation
Refers to the actual production of speech sounds. It refers to the child's ability to move the articulators in the mouth as opposed to the ability to plan an utterance in the brain.

Articulators
Refers to the moving parts in the mouth – tongue, lips, soft palate and the sphincter linking the oral and nasal cavities.

Assistant

Classroom
The classroom assistant or 'special needs assistant' refers to individuals specifically employed to work in the classroom with children with special needs. In some cases these assistants are allocated to specific children. In other cases they are generic workers and work with groups of children for a variety of purposes.

Speech and language therapy
Speech and language therapy assistants are employed by speech and language therapy departments and work alongside or under the super-

vision of therapists, carrying out programmes for individual children or groups of children as required. They may work in the classroom or in the clinic/health centre.

Augmentative communication

Augmentative communication refers to different systems that can be introduced to augment or enhance the child's communication skills. These may be manual, sign systems, technological aids or communication boards. It is important that these only ever supplement the child's skills and are never intended to replace them.

Children Act (1989)

The Children Act draws together all the existing legislation designed to protect the rights of the child. It emphasises the role played by the family and stresses the need to work through the family in all but the most exceptional of cases. It also has a lot to say about the role of children in care and highlights the need for the recognition of the needs of children with developmental and medical difficulties. It stresses the need for inter-agency collaboration particularly between social, health and educational agencies.

Code of Practice

Department for Education guidance published in 1994 for children with special educational needs to which schools, health authorities and social services have a statutory duty to 'have regard to'.

Comprehension

Verbal

Verbal comprehension refers to the child's ability to comprehend the spoken word. Therapists always assess verbal comprehension to ensure that this is not at the root of the child's difficulties. Such assessments are often very structured in order to cut out extraneous clues which might help the child answer the questions.

Non-verbal

Non-verbal comprehension refers to all the other ways in which children use the context to understand what someone is saying. Typically this would be pointing and eye-pointing to requested objects, facial expressions, gestures etc. It is very important to establish to what extent children are using such clues.

Conductive hearing loss
A temporary and often fluctuating hearing loss associated with infection
or blockage in the middle ear – i.e. immediately inside the ear drum.

Content of language
We speak of the form, content and use of language. Content refers to the
child's intended meaning. Does the child have a range of such meanings
– requesting, denying etc. – at his disposal? If not, this may be a focus of
intervention.

Criterion referenced tests/procedures
These are assessments which have been developed from what we know
about development using the scientific literature. They have not been
standardised on a lot of children (see standardised tests) and we do not
use them to obtain standardised scores or age equivalent scores.

Derbyshire Language Scheme (DLS)
A programme designed for use with children acquiring the early stages of
language. It emphasises the need to assess verbal comprehension prior to
commencing intervention. It introduces the concept of the 'information
carrying word' into the speech and language therapist's vocabulary.
Similarly, when they speak of 'word levels' this too comes from the DLS.
It promotes the child's functional use of language and encourages the
child's ability to take control of language activities through role reversal.

Developmental delay
This means that development in one or more areas is following the normal
developmental pattern but at a slower rate than would be expected for the
child's chronological age. Usually contrasted with a disorder, a term which
suggests that the development is not following a normal developmental
pattern.

Developmental norm
Children acquire different skills at different ages and there may be
considerable variation between individual children. Nonetheless it is
possible to speak of an average range for each skill. These are sometimes
referred to as developmental norms. Children falling outside such norms
are often considered to be in need of additional support.

Differential diagnosis

The process by which the doctor or therapist ascertains the nature of the child's problems by excluding other conditions.

Dysfluency

This is a term used to describe non-fluent or hesitant speech. Also known as stammering or stuttering.

Dyspraxia

Dyspraxia is a diagnostic term intended for use with children who have difficulties planning what they intend to say. The effect is highly unintelligible speech. The children can often produce sounds in isolation but they become increasingly difficult to understand as they try to put the sounds into words and then into sentences.

Edinburgh Articulation Test

A test comprising a set of pictures designed to elicit a range of speech sounds within words.

Education Acts

1944

The concept of children with speech and language difficulties in the absence of more pronounced developmental difficulties first included in legislation.

1981

The Formal Assessment (FA) procedure first introduced. Increased emphasis on children being integrated into mainstream classrooms rather than being placed in special schools or units.

1988

Local management of schools introduced.

1993

Draft code of Practice introduced.

1994

The Code of Practice.

Expressive Language

See Language Production.

Form of language
We speak of the form, content and use of language. Form refers to the outward aspects of language – the sounds, the syntax and the way in which words are modified to change their meanings, e.g. plural or verb endings.

Grammar
Often seen as meaning the same as 'syntax', grammar refers to the way in which words can be combined.

Hanen Early Language Parent Programme
A very carefully designed programme developed in Canada but coming to increasing prominence in the UK. It is designed to promote the communication skills and language development of young children. The parent rather than the child is the focus of the programme.

Information Carrying words
Words which carry key imformation within an utterance. See also Derbyshire Language Scheme.

Integration
Integration is a term first introduced into law in 1981 to refer to the need for children with special needs to be kept within their mainstream classroom to mix with their peers etc. Often easier to talk about than to carry out. The children's needs should be carefully considered in each case.

Lancashire Judgement
This was a legal judgement made in 1989 which suggested that provision for the speech and language difficulties of school-aged children should fall within the remit of the Department for Education rather than the National Health Service. This has been contested and the responsibility for the provision for these children continues to be a matter for discussion.

Language

Production
Production refers to the child's capacity to express herself. Conventionally this refers to speech but it can equally apply to the child's use of augmentative systems.

Comprehension
See verbal comprehension above. It is always important to be aware of how a child makes use of what they understand of the non linguistic context to help them understand what others are saying.

Delay
This is a term used to suggest that the child's language level is equivalent to that of a younger child and is usually contrasted with disorder. Recent research work suggests that the majority of children with language impairments fit into this category. It is probably most widely used up to the early school years. Thereafter the child's experience is likely to mean that they will have very little in common with a child whose tested language levels are similar.

Disorder
This term is contrasted with delay (see above) and suggests that there is something abnormal about the child's language development above and beyond the delay. Such conditions become much more apparent as the child gets older.

Impairment
This is a generic term referring to all clinical levels of language difficulty. It suggests that there is something structurally different about the way the children respond to language which distinguishes them from 'normal' language learners.

Units
Children with severe language impairments are sometimes placed in language units. Here they are provided with specialist teaching and therapy. Such units are usually set within mainstream schools. Sometimes they are referred to as language classes.

Living Language
A programme to help promote language – and especially vocabulary development.

Local Management of Schools (LMS)
This came in following the 1988 Education Act and gives schools their own budgets. This inevitably has implications for those children with special needs.

Mainstream school
Local state funded primary and secondary schools. They are usually contrasted with 'special schools'.

Metaphon therapy
A programme developed for the remediation of children with difficulties acquiring the rules of speech development (phonology).

Nuffield Dyspraxia Programme
A programme developed for the remediation of children with difficulties coordinating the motor movements associated with speech production.

Phonology
Phonology refers to the rules which allow children to perceive and produce the differences between sounds in a highly regular manner. These rules are usually acquired in the first three or four years of life although the speed at which they can mark these differences varies considerably.

Pragmatics
Pragmatics refers to the child's ability to use language in context. When we talk about pragmatics we are always interested in the speaker and the listener, in what is said and the way that it is perceived.

Raw score
This is a term used when counting the number of correct responses on a standardised test. It is contrasted with the standard score which refers to the child's score compared to what would be expected for the child's age.

Receptive Language
See Verbal Comprehension.

Semantics
This refers to the meaning conveyed by vocabulary and the grammatical structures that the child uses.

Special School
Schools funded by the Local Educational Authority, or independently, designed to provide for children whose needs may not be met within a mainstream school.

Speech
Speech is the meaningful articulation of sounds.

Standardised tests
Standardised tests are tests developed on a representative sample of subjects. It is then possible to compare a given child's response to the test in question with that original sample. This allows us to calculate a number of ways of describing that child's skills – standard score, age equivalent, percentile rank etc.

Standard score
The single most important score derived from a standardised test, this allows us to express the child's performance in terms of where it comes relative to the group of children on whom the test was originally developed. The average on such tests is normally taken as 100 and the child's performance may be expressed as a function of the number of 'standard deviations' from the average (usually 15 points) or as a single score.

Statement of special educational needs
A legal document to which parents and professionals contribute. This describes the child's special educational needs and the resources and provision required to meet those needs.

Support teacher
A teacher specialising in learning support of any kind. They may be based in a single school or in a team which then takes on work with children in a number of schools. Such teachers may have additional qualifications.

Syntax
See Grammar.

Use of language
We speak of the form, content and use of language. Use of language is comparable to the term pragmatics (see above) and refers to the child's ability to use language in context.

Index

AFASIC 3, 4, 11, 13, 16, 119, 135, 139–146, 157–158

age equivalent score 42, 43, 61, 78, 89

anoxia 36, 95,

articulation *see* speech

assessments 34, 35, 39
  formal 40, 41–45, 67, 89
  informal 40–41

assistant 93, 113, 124

attention *see* listening

augmentative communication 82, 109, 118, 131–132, 137

autism 11, 83

behaviour 101–102, 110

bilingualism 24–25, 37, 42, 75

birth history 53, 97

blood tests 55

brain
  development 32
  damage 12, 77, 98
  scans 56, 77

Bus Story 43

cerebral palsy 79

child development centre 53, 56, 57, 107, 120

chromosomes 55

cleft palate 24

Clinical Evaluation of Language Fundamentals (CELF–R) 42, 43

clumsy 66

Code of Practice 35, 58, 104, 106, 107, 113, 147–152

cognitive skills 28

coordination of speech *see* speech

community clinics 107, 109

comprehension
  verbal 9, 22–23, 41, 47–48, 81, 90, 94, 118, 123, 127, 138
  non verbal 6,

Derbyshire Language Scheme 43, 44, 127–128, 130, 132

developmental checks 5, 34, 52

developmental delay 37

diagnosis 37, 74

doctors – gp 5, 9, 34, 35, 37, 52
  paediatrician 5, 52–57, 76

Down's Syndrome 55, 79, 90, 95

dysfluency 86–87

dysphasia 77, 81

dyspraxia 12, 13, 25, 77, 84–86, 103, 129, 141

eating 53, 68, 92

echolalia 82

Edinburgh Articulation Test 49

Education acts
  1981 56, 104, 112
  1993 104–107, 147, 153

Educational Psychologist 2, 52, 57–61, 105, 106, 137

epilepsy 56, 98

expression 44, 48–49, 81, 94, 123, 138

family history 37

feeding *see* eating

Fragile X Syndrome 55, 95,

genetic factors 95
grammar 23, 28–29, 43, 48, 80
group speech and language therapy 125

Hanen Early Language Parent Programme 130–131
health visitors 5, 9, 34, 35, 37, 52, 53, 91
hearing 5, 21, 26, 53
hearing loss 26, 78, 90, 95–96, 103, 109

individual speech and language therapy 125
information carrying words (ICW) 22, 44, 127
integration 101, 110
intelligence quotient (IQ) 59, 60
Invalid Children's Aid Nationwide 3, 135–139

language
delay 11, 79–81, 133
disorder 11, 79–81, 112
impairment 11, 78–79, 81–84, 90, 98, 112, 122, 140, 154
unit 14, 15, 75, 108–112, 115, 140, 144
Learning support service 113–114
lexical syntactic disorder 83–84
listening 21–22, 36, 41, 45–46, 96, 138
literacy 92, 102–103, 115, 133–134
Living Language 128, 130, 132
local education authority (LEA) 7, 61, 105–7, 112, 113, 138, 150–152, 153–156
Lowe and Costello Symbolic Play Test 43, 46

Mainstream school 75, 78, 93, 108, 111, 112–115, 121, 138

Makaton see augmentative communication
memory 23, 27,
Metaphon 49, 129
Motor skills 11, 37, 53, 62–65, 71–72

National Curriculum 31, 39, 40, 50, 61, 78, 109, 112, 132, 142, 145, 149
neuro developmental examination 54
nondirective therapy 130
non verbal skills 28, 36, 60–61
normal nonfluency 26
note in lieu 155–156
Nuffield Dyspraxia Programme 49, 128–129

Occupational Therapist, 2, 52, 53, 65–73
oral examination 49–50

Paget Gorman
  Signing System *see*
  augmentaive
  communication
Parents 4–17, 36,
  98–100,
  123–124,
  136–139, 140–
  141, 147–156
performance *see* non
  verbal skills
phonology *see* speech
phonological
  disorders 84–86,
  141
Phonological
  Assessment of
  Child Speech 49,
Physiotherapist 2, 52,
  53, 62–65,
play 27–28, 40–41,
  43, 46–47, 53,
  59, 68
Pragmatics Profile 51
primary language
  impairment *see*
  language
  impairment

reading *see* literacy
receptive language *see*
  comprehension
residential school
  111–116
Reynell
  Developmental

Language Scales
  42, 43

secondary language
  impairment *see*
  language
  impairment
semantics 29, 48
semantic pragmatic
  disorder 82–83,
  141
signing *see*
  augmentative
  communication
social factors 98–100
social interaction 35,
  39, 44, 50, 99
South Tyneside
  Assessment of
  Child Speech 49
special educational
  needs tribunal
  153–155
special school 9, 78,
  104, 115–116,
  135–138
special needs
  coordinator
  (SENCO) 113, 149
specific language
  impairment *see*
  language
  impairment
speech and language
  therapy 5, 7, 8,
  15, 16, 22,
  34–51, 53, 57,

74, 77, 107,
  117–134, 135,
  137–139, 144
speech 24–36,
  49–51, 83,
  84–87, 92, 141
stammering *see* fluency
standard score 41, 46,
  89
standardised tests *see*
  formal assessments
Statement of
  Educational Need
  16, 57, 104–108,
  147–156,
  152–153, 165–
  167
stuttering *see* fluency
symbolic play *see* play
syntax *see* grammar

tests *see* formal
  assessments
Test of Reception of
  Grammar (TROG)
  43

use of language 29,
  30, 48, 50–51, 82

vocabulary 23, 38,
  48, 91, 128, 138
voice *see* speech

word finding
    difficulties 44, 118
writing *see* literacy

Children with Autism
Diagnosis and Interventions to Meet Their Needs

Colwyn Trevarthen, Kenneth J. Aitken, Despina Papoudi
and Jacqueline Z. Robarts
1996 256 pages ISBN 1 85302 314 0 pb

Approaching the condition of autism from many perspectives, the authors make a comprehensive study of the disorder, balancing theory with practice, and presenting a clear picture of what it means to be autistic, and what can be done to improve the capabilities of the autistic child. They consider

- the historical descriptions, explanations and recognition of the condition
- the symptons and causes
- the classification of autism and related conditions such as Asperger's syndrome, including details of the latest diagnostic systems and they examine methods of
- communicating with autistic children
- helping them to communicate as fully as possible.

Calling on recent developmental research and new data on the communication and emotions of autistic children, and new findings on brain development, they examine the results of recent intervention trials to provide a wealth of information that will be helpful for parents, caregivers and those planning education and care.

Colwyn Trevarthen is Professor of Child Psychology and Psychobiology at Edinburgh University.

CONTENTS: 1.Introduction. 2.What is Autism? 3.What Autism is Not. 4.How Many Autistic Children? 5.What Causes Autism? 6.Where Development Goes Astray. 7.Communicating and Playing with an Autistic Child. 8.What Can Be Done? 9.Music Making to Aid Communication. 10.Recommendations for Education of Autistic Children. Bibliography. Glossary.

Jessica Kingsley Publishers
116 Pentonville Road, London N1 9JB

Children with Language Impairments
An Introduction
Morag L. Donaldson
144 pages ISBN 1 85302 313 2 pb

There are many ways of defining and categorising language and communication disorders, and this introduction examines:

- definitions of language impairments in children
- categorising language impairments
- methods of diagnosis and assessment
- related or accompanying problems
- testing methods
- strategies for intervention.

Examining the prevalence of language disorders in children, the book is an important summary of current awareness of language impairments in children. The book offers advice on assessment methods and intervention, and provides a detailed glossary of the most important terminology used.

CONTENTS: 1 Introduction. *1.1 Reflecting on language difficulties. 1.2 Language and communication. 1.3 Language, spoken language and speech. 1.4 Disorder, disability, impairment, delay and deviance. 1.5 Standards of comparison.* 2 Categorising language Impairments. *2.1 The medical approach. 2.2 The linguistic approach. 2.3 Combining the medical and linguistic taxonomies. 2.4 Children with Secondary Language Impairments. 2.5 Children with Specific Language Impairments. 2.5 Overview and Implications.* 3 Prevalence of language Impairments in children. *3.1 Prevalence Studies. 3.2 Prevalence Rates. 3.3 Gender. 3.4 Social Class 3.5 Intelligence. 3.6 Behaviour Problems 3.7 Overview and Implications.* 4. Prognosis for children with language disorders. *4.1 Stability of language Impairments. 4.2 Prognosis for reading abilities. 4.3 Prognosis for intelligence. 4.4 Prognosis for Socio-Emotional and Behaviour problems. 4.5 Overview and Implications.* 5. Assessing language disorders. *5.1 Functions of assessment. 5.2 Contexts of assessment. 5.3 Standardized tests. 5.4 Naturalistic observations. 5.5 Non-standardized elicitations. 5.6 Overview and Implications.* 6. Approaches to Intervention. *6.1 Issues of intervention. 6.2 Goals of intervention. 6.3 Intervention techniques. 6.4 Agents of intervention. 6.5 Settings of intervention. 6.6 Overview and Implications.* 7. In Conclusion. References. Glossary. Index.

Dr Morag L. Donaldson works at the Edinburgh Centre for Research in Child Development, University of Edinburgh.

Jessica Kingsley Publishers
116 Pentonville Road, London N1 9JB

Language Development in Children with Special Needs
Performative Communication

Irene Johansson
Translated by Eva Thomas
1994 160 pages ISBN 1 85302 241 1 pb

'a very practical and accessible book, supported by relevant theory, which should be useful to parents, carers and other professionals.'

– Mencap News

'A range of activities aimed at developing a 'structured conversation' with the child are offered, where it is clearly indicated as to what the parent should say or do in order to proactively encourage and listen to the child.'

– Nursery World

Irene Johansson is Professor at the Department of Linguistics, Umea University. **Eva Thomas** is a Speech and Language Therapist, Eastbourne Health Authority

Jessica Kingsley Publishers
116 Pentonville Road, London N1 9JB

Young Adults with Special Needs
Assessment, Law and Practice – Caught in the Acts
John Friel
1995 140 pages ISBN 1 85302 231 4 pb

'This new book is a comprehensive, yet commendably condensed, over-view of the situation...it is sure to find a place on the bookshelves of parents, FE College staff and care agencies. I would like to think that LEA's and the Further Education Funding Council will also use the book to inform their thinking and practice in this important area... This book, and a sympathetic lawyer will help to guide us through the laby-rinth...should become an essential *vade mecum* for all involved with young adults who have special needs.'

– Down Syndrome Association

Reviewed with *Children with Special Needs*

'...both books will be relevant to all who work with children and young adults with special needs...they are both superbly produced, clearly and accessibly laid out and undoubtedly a key source of information and guidance for anyone responsible for supporting individuals with special needs.'

– Young People Now

John Friel is a barrister-at-law at Grays Inn specialising in work relating to children with special needs.

Jessica Kingsley Publishers
116 Pentonville Road, London N1 9JB

Children with Special Needs
Assessment, Law and Practice – Caught in the Act, 3rd edition

John Friel

1995 240 pages ISBN 1 85302 280 2 pb

Review of the third edition, and *Young Adults with Special Needs*

'…both books will be relevant to all who work with children and young adults with special needs…they are both superbly produced, clearly and accessibly laid out and undoubtedly a key source of information and guidance for anyone responsible for supporting individuals with special needs.'

– Young People Now

Reviews of previous editions

'This book provides valuable assistance for parents in what is often an uneven struggle with education authorities over the vital area of children's education.'

– Dyslexia Contact

'Such a book should prove an essential guide for parents and educators of children with special educational needs and the legal procedure for obtaining the education they need.'

– Disability News

John Friel is a barrister-at-law at Grays Inn specialising in work relating to children with special needs.

Jessica Kingsley Publishers
116 Pentonville Road, London N1 9JB